Adverse Effects of Psychotropic Treatments

Editor

RAJNISH MAGO

PSYCHIATRIC CLINICS
OF NORTH AMERICA

www.psych.theclinics.com

September 2016 • Volume 39 • Number 3

ELSEVIER

1600 John F. Kennedy Boulevard • Suite 1800 • Philadelphia, Pennsylvania, 19103-2899

http://www.theclinics.com

PSYCHIATRIC CLINICS OF NORTH AMERICA Volume 39, Number 3
September 2016 ISSN 0193-953X, ISBN-13: 978-0-323-46265-5

Editor: Lauren Boyle
Developmental Editor: Kristen Helm

Psychiatric Clinics of North America (ISSN 0193-953X) is published quarterly by Elsevier Inc., 360 Park Avenue South, New York, NY 10010-1710. Months of issue are March, June, September, and December. Business and Editorial Offices: 1600 John F. Kennedy Blvd., Suite 1800, Philadelphia, PA 19103-2899. Periodicals postage paid at New York, NY and additional mailing offices. Subscription prices are $300.00 per year (US individuals), $598.00 per year (US institutions), $100.00 per year (US students/residents), $365.00 per year (Canadian individuals), $455.00 per year (international individuals), $753.00 per year (Canadian & international institutions), and $220.00 per year (Canadian & international students/residents). Foreign air speed delivery is included in all *Clinics'* subscription prices. All prices are subject to change without notice. POSTMASTER: Send address changes to *Psychiatric Clinics of North America*, Elsevier Health Sciences Division, Subscription Customer Service, 3251 Riverport Lane, Maryland Heights, MO 63043. **Customer Service: 1-800-654-2452 (US). From outside the United States, call 1-314-447-8871. Fax: 1-314-447-8029. E-mail: journalscustomerservice-usa@elsevier.com (for print support)** and **journalsonline support-usa@elsevier.com (for online support).**

Reprints. For copies of 100 or more, of articles in this publication, please contact the Commercial Reprints Department, Elsevier Inc., 360 Park Avenue South, New York, New York 10010-1710. Tel.: 212-633-3874, Fax: 212-633-3820, E-mail: reprints@elsevier.com.

Psychiatric Clinics of North America is covered in *MEDLINE/PubMed (Index Medicus), Current Contents/Social and Behavioral Sciences, Social Science Citation Index, Embase/Excerpta Medica,* and PsycINFO.

Contributors

EDITOR

RAJNISH MAGO, MD
Editor-in-Chief, Simpleandpractical.com, Philadelphia, Pennsylvania

AUTHORS

ANDREW R. ALKIS, MD
Chief Resident, Department of Psychiatry and Neurobehavioral Sciences, University of Virginia, Charlottesville, Virginia

CHITTARANJAN ANDRADE, MD
Professor and Head, Department of Psychopharmacology, National Institute of Mental Health and Neurosciences, Bangalore, India

SHYAM SUNDAR ARUMUGHAM, MD, DNB
Associate Professor, Department of Psychiatry, National Institute of Mental Health and Neurosciences, Bangalore, India

DAVID A. BRENT, MD
Academic Chief, Child and Adolescent Psychiatry; Professor of Psychiatry; Endowed Chair, Suicide Studies, University of Pittsburgh School of Medicine, Pittsburgh, Pennsylvania

E. CABRINA CAMPBELL, MD
Associate Professor, Department of Psychiatry, Perelman School of Medicine, University of Pennsylvania, Corporal Michael J. Crescenz Veterans Affairs Medical Center, Philadelphia, Pennsylvania

STANLEY N. CAROFF, MD
Emeritus Professor, Department of Psychiatry, Perelman School of Medicine, University of Pennsylvania, Philadelphia, Pennsylvania

ANITA H. CLAYTON, MD
Professor and Chair, Department of Psychiatry and Neurobehavioral Sciences, University of Virginia, Charlottesville, Virginia

KARL DOGHRAMJI, MD
Professor of Psychiatry, Neurology, and Medicine; Program Director, Fellowship in Sleep Medicine, Department of Psychiatry and Human Behavior; Medical Director, Jefferson Sleep Disorders Center, Sidney Kimmel Medical College, Thomas Jefferson University, Philadelphia, Pennsylvania

CARRIE L. ERNST, MD
Associate Professor of Psychiatry, Departments of Psychiatry and Medical Education, Icahn School of Medicine at Mount Sinai, New York, New York

MARLENE P. FREEMAN, MD
Associate Director, Perinatal and Reproductive Psychiatry, Department of Psychiatry, Massachusetts General Hospital, Boston, Massachusetts

JOSEPH F. GOLDBERG, MD
Clinical Professor, Department of Psychiatry, Icahn School of Medicine at Mount Sinai, New York, New York

CHARLOTTE S. HOGAN, MD
Clinical Fellow, Department of Psychiatry, Massachusetts General Hospital, Boston, Massachusetts

WILLIAM C. JANGRO, DO
Assistant Professor of Psychiatry; Associate Director, Adult Residency Training Program, Department of Psychiatry and Human Behavior, Sidney Kimmel Medical College, Thomas Jefferson University, Philadelphia, Pennsylvania

RAJNISH MAGO, MD
Editor-in-Chief, Simpleandpractical.com, Philadelphia, Pennsylvania

NISHANT B. PARIKH, MD
Resident Physician, Department of Psychiatry and Neurobehavioral Sciences, University of Virginia, Charlottesville, Virginia

EESHA SHARMA, MD
Assistant Professor, Department of Psychiatry, King George's Medical University, Lucknow, India

MICHAEL E. THASE, MD
Professor of Psychiatry, Perelman School of Medicine, University of Pennsylvania, Corporal Michael J. Crescenz Veterans Affairs Medical Center, Philadelphia, Pennsylvania

JAGADISHA THIRTHALLI, MD
Professor, Department of Psychiatry, National Institute of Mental Health and Neurosciences, Bangalore, India

JENNIFER G. VOTTA, DO
Resident Physician, Department of Psychiatry and Neurobehavioral Sciences, University of Virginia, Charlottesville, Virginia

Contents

> Adverse effects are common, bothersome, and a leading cause of discontinuation of treatment. The methodology for evaluating adverse effects of medications has been greatly neglected, however, especially in comparison to the methodology for assessment of efficacy of medications. Existing methods for assessment and reporting of adverse effects have important limitations leading to lack of much-needed data related to adverse effects. Lastly, there is little systematic research into management of most adverse effects. A series of recommendations are made in this article about how to improve identification, assessment, reporting, and management of adverse effects.

> Adverse effects from psychiatric drugs can profoundly influence treatment adherence and outcomes. Good care involves addressing adverse effects no differently than any other component of treatment. Knowledge about adverse effect assessment and management fosters a proper context that helps clinicians not sacrifice a drug's potential therapeutic benefits because of greater concerns about its tolerability. This article provides an overview of basic concepts related to the assessment and management of suspected adverse effects from psychotropic drugs. Key points are discussed regarding clinical, pharmacogenetic, pharmacokinetic, and pharmacodynamic risk factors for treatment-emergent adverse effects, alongside recommendations for their systematic assessment.

> The development of drugs to treat psychosis is a fascinating nexus for understanding mechanisms underlying disorders of mind and movement. Although the risk of drug-induced extrapyramidal syndromes has been mitigated by the acceptance of less potent dopamine antagonists, expansive marketing and off-label use has increased the number of susceptible people who may be at risk for these neurologic effects. Clinicians need to be familiar with advances in diagnosis and management, which are reviewed herein. A better understanding of drug-induced effects on the motor circuit may improve patient safety, enhance antipsychotic effectiveness, and provide insights into mechanisms underlying antipsychotic activity in parallel brain circuits.

Serotonin reuptake inhibitors (SRIs) increase the risk of abnormal bleeding by lowering platelet serotonin and hence the efficiency of platelet-driven hemostasis; by increasing gastric acidity and possibly gastric ulceration; and by other mechanisms. The upper gastrointestinal tract is the commonest site of SRI-related abnormal bleeding; bleeding at this location may be increased by concurrent nonsteroidal anti-inflammatory drug therapy and by treatment with antiplatelet or anticoagulant drugs. Bleeding at this location may be reduced by concurrent administration of acid-suppressing drugs.

Sexual functioning is important to assess in patients with psychiatric illness as both the condition and associated treatment may contribute to sexual dysfunction (SD). Antidepressant medications, mood stabilizers, antipsychotics, and antianxiety agents may be associated with SD related to drug mechanism of action. Sexual adverse effects may be related to genetic risk factors, impact on neurotransmitters and hormones, and psychological elements. Effective strategies to manage medication-induced sexual dysfunction are initial choice of a drug unlikely to cause SD, switching to a different medication, and adding an antidote to reverse SD. Appropriate interventions should be determined on a clinical case-by-case basis.

Management of bipolar disorder during pregnancy often involves medications with potential adverse effects, including risks to the mother and fetus. Although some specifics are known, many medications continue to have incompletely characterized reproductive safety profiles. Women with bipolar disorder who are planning pregnancy face challenging decisions about their treatment; careful risk-benefit discussions are necessary. With the goal of further informing these discussions, this article reviews the data currently available regarding medication safety in the management of bipolar disorder during pregnancy, with specific attention to lithium, valproic acid, lamotrigine, carbamazepine, and antipsychotic medications.

Over the past decades, several adjunctive therapies have been introduced for treatment-resistant depression (TRD), and these strategies have ebbed and flowed in popularity. Currently, adjunctive therapy with the second-generation antipsychotics (SGAs) is most commonly used by psychiatrists. Four SGAs are FDA approved for indications related to TRD (aripiprazole, brexpiprazole, olanzapine, and quetiapine extended release); some evidence also supports use of risperidone and ziprasidone as adjunctive therapies. This article briefly reviews the role of adjunctive therapy with SGAs in contemporary algorithms for TRD, considering both the evidence of benefit and the adverse effects.

Psychotropic medications such as antidepressants, antipsychotics, stimulants, and benzodiazepines are widely prescribed. Most of these medications are thought to exert their effects through modulation of various monoamines as well as interactions with receptors such as histamine and muscarinic cholinergic receptors. Through these interactions, psychotropics can also have a significant impact on sleep physiology, resulting in both beneficial and adverse effects on sleep.

We review the evidence that antidepressants either increase or decrease the risk for suicidal ideation and behavior in adolescents. Meta-analyses of randomized clinical trials (RCTs) indicate a small increased risk for suicidal events in adolescents and young adults, but a protective effect in older adults. In contrast, pharmacoepidemiologic studies show a protective effect across the life span. Explanations for occurrence of suicidal events in younger patients and for the apparent contradiction between RCT and pharmacoepidemiologic studies are offered. Guidance for clinicians is provided on explaining the risk-benefit ratio of antidepressants and how to monitor and attenuate for suicidal risk.

Electroconvulsive therapy (ECT) is an effective treatment commonly used for depression and other major psychiatric disorders. We discuss potential adverse effects (AEs) associated with ECT and strategies for their prevention and management. Common acute AEs include headache, nausea, myalgia, and confusion; these are self-limiting and are managed symptomatically. Serious but uncommon AEs include cardiovascular, pulmonary, and cerebrovascular events; these may be minimized with screening for risk factors and by physiologic monitoring. Although most cognitive AEs of ECT are short-lasting, troublesome retrograde amnesia may rarely persist. Modifications of and improvements in treatment techniques minimize cognitive and other AEs.

PSYCHIATRIC CLINICS OF NORTH AMERICA

RELATED INTEREST

Primary Care: Clinics in Office Practice, June 2016 (Vol. 43, No. 2)
Psychiatric Care in Primary Care Practice
Janet R. Albers, *Editor*
Available at http://www.primarycare.theclinics.com/

Preface

The Neglected Side of Suffering

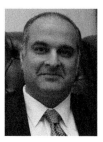

Rajnish Mago, MD
Editor

Adverse effects of psychotropic medications have substantial impact on patient suffering, on nonadherence to treatment, and ultimately, on the success of treatment. Yet, somewhat surprisingly, adverse effects have been considerably neglected in research and in publications. Thus, this issue of the *Psychiatric Clinics of North America* should be a welcome addition to the literature.

The first article in this issue is a "call to action" that aims to draw attention to the importance of adverse effects. It highlights some of the many problems related to how adverse effects are identified and assessed, how patients are educated about adverse effects, and the relative paucity of research about their prevention and management. A series of recommendations aimed at beginning to remedy these problems is also made.

This is followed by an article by Goldberg and Ernst that provides an insightful discussion of the complexity of how clinical and pharmacogenetic factors contribute to the incidence and severity of adverse effects of psychotropic medications. It also provides valuable clinical guidance on several issues, like how to counsel patients about adverse effects, how to differentiate adverse effects from symptoms of the illness, and so on.

The articles that follow are up-to-date reviews of the literature, all by leading experts, on some of the most important topics related to adverse effects of mental health treatments.

Though second-generation antipsychotics have reduced the incidence of extrapyramidal and related adverse effects, these continue to be significant problems for some patients. Clinicians, therefore, need to be well-versed in their identification and management. Caroff and Campbell provide us with a pithy, up-to-date review of dystonia, parkinsonism, akathisia, catatonia, neuroleptic malignant syndrome, and tardive dyskinesia that will be helpful to clinicians.

Andrade and Sharma succinctly review the state-of-the-art on abnormal bleeding that can be caused by antidepressant medications. They also summarize current

Psychiatr Clin N Am 39 (2016) ix–x
http://dx.doi.org/10.1016/j.psc.2016.06.001
0193-953X/16/$ – see front matter © 2016 Elsevier Inc. All rights reserved.

knowledge on how concomitant medications and illness can moderate the risk of bleeding with antidepressants, and provide recommendations in how to manage this increased risk.

In their comprehensive review, Clayton and colleagues discuss a wide variety of issues related to sexual dysfunction associated not only with antidepressant medications (including the most recently introduced ones) but also with other psychotropic medications.

In recent years, many publications have addressed the risks associated with use of antidepressant medications during pregnancy. The article by Hogan and Freeman, on the other hand, summarizes current knowledge on the potential adverse effects on pregnancy of other medications—those that are often used to treat persons with bipolar disorder, including mood stabilizers and antipsychotics. Clinicians who treat women of childbearing age who suffer from bipolar disorder will find this review very helpful.

While second-generation antipsychotics generally have a more favorable profile in terms of extrapyramidal symptoms, they can be associated with significant risks of akathisia and metabolic syndrome. These second-generation antipsychotics are now widely used as adjuncts to antidepressants. The article by Thase focuses specifically on the potential adverse effects of second-generation antipsychotics when used as adjuncts and provides a balanced discussion of risk-benefit considerations.

Doghramji and Jangro have reviewed the literature on a neglected but clinically important topic—the potential adverse effects of a variety of psychotropic medications on sleep. Their article should make clinicians more aware of the possibility that the psychotropic medication(s) being prescribed may be adversely affecting sleep.

Next, the review by Brent helps us to understand the otherwise confusing data on the potential relationship between antidepressant medications and increased risk of suicidal ideation or behavior and helps the reader make sense of the confusing data. Importantly, he provides clinical guidance regarding how to reduce and manage this risk.

Patients frequently have concerns about the potential adverse effects of electroconvulsive therapy. In the final article of this issue, Andrade and colleagues review the potential adverse effects of this important and still relevant treatment modality. Even clinicians who themselves don't administer electroconvulsive therapy need to have accurate information about these potential risks in order to be able to discuss them with patients and families.

I am confident that the articles in this issue significantly add to and update the literature on adverse effects of treatments for mental disorders. My hope is that it will encourage the field to pay greater attention to the problem of adverse effects, both in terms of research and in clinical practice, eventually leading to better outcomes for our patients.

Rajnish Mago, MD
Simpleandpractical.com
210 West Rittenhouse Square
Suite 404
Philadelphia, PA 19103, USA

E-mail address:
mago@simpleandpractical.com

Adverse Effects of Psychotropic Medications

A Call to Action

Rajnish Mago, MD

KEYWORDS

- Adverse effects • Side effects • Psychiatric medications • Psychotropic medications
- Clinical trials • Rating scales • CONSORT

KEY POINTS

- Clinicians need to fully appreciate the extent to which nonadherence is a pervasive problem that vitiates the effectiveness of psychotropic medications.
- Adverse effects need to be viewed not as a necessary and unavoidable price to be paid for the benefits of treatment but as a major cause of suffering and nonadherence that need to be energetically prevented, reduced, and managed.
- The methodology for identification, assessment, and reporting of adverse events in clinical trials needs to be improved and standardized.
- A substantial increase in research into management of various adverse effects is needed. Many strategies to reduce and manage adverse effects, however, are already available but need to be used more often to reduce nonadherence to medications.

Adverse effects (a more appropriate term than *side effects*) of psychotropic medications are often viewed by clinicians as the unfortunate, unwanted, and perhaps inevitable accompaniments of the benefits of these medications. To the persons taking these medications, however, the distress caused by these adverse effects is as important as that caused by the symptoms of the disorder being treated. Patients are put in the unfortunate position of having to weigh the benefits of the medications against the burden of adverse effects. Given how important adverse effects are to patients, and often to their families, and given the central role they play in nonadherence to medication, it is astonishing how little attention has been paid to the identification and management of these adverse effects.

Disclosure: Grant/Research Support (to Thomas Jefferson University, with Dr R. Mago as the Principal Investigator): Alkermes, Inc; Allergan, Plc (formerly Forest Research Institute); Genomind, Inc; and Takeda Pharmaceuticals U.S.A.; Consultant: Allergan, Plc (formerly Forest Laboratories); Genomind, Inc; Lundbeck, LLC; and Otsuka America Pharmaceutical, Inc.
Simpleandpractical.com, 210 West Rittenhouse Square, Suite 404, Philadelphia, PA 19103, USA
E-mail address: mago@simpleandpractical.com

Psychiatr Clin N Am 39 (2016) 361–373
http://dx.doi.org/10.1016/j.psc.2016.04.005
0193-953X/16/$ – see front matter © 2016 Elsevier Inc. All rights reserved.

I start by reviewing some of the reasons why adverse effects are so important, then discuss the various problems faced with regard to adverse effects, and, finally, propose a plan of action to address some of those problems.

ADVERSE EFFECTS ARE BOTH COMMON AND BOTHERSOME

A great majority of persons taking a psychotropic medication have 1 or more adverse effects of that medication. Are most of these adverse effects, isolated, mild, and of little clinical significance? In a survey of patients prescribed a selective serotonin reuptake inhibitor (SSRI), 52% of patients reported that they had had 3 or more adverse effects, and 55% reported that they had had at least 1 adverse effect that was either "a lot" or "extremely" bothersome.[1,2]

The drug-placebo differences for the most common adverse events occurring in clinical trials of psychotropic medications, as noted in the prescribing information for these medications, are shown in **Table 1**. The numbers show that adverse effects occur in a substantial number of patients who take these medications. Individual adverse events are reported by 3% to 39% more patients on the medication versus on placebo. These numbers are probably an underestimate of the true incidence of these adverse events because in clinical trials adverse events are identified mainly or entirely based on spontaneous reporting.

ADVERSE EFFECTS OFTEN LEAD TO DISCONTINUATION OF TREATMENT

A majority of persons prescribed a psychotropic medication soon stop taking it, vitiating the effectiveness of treatment. For example, in 1 study, 28% of patients completely discontinued taking any antidepressant within the first 3 months after starting on an antidepressant; in addition, others switched the antidepressant and more discontinued the medication later in treatment.[3]

Why do they discontinue the medications? The most common reason for discontinuing or switching an SSRI within the first 3 months is adverse effects.[3] Similar findings were more recently reported in patients treated with reboxetine or citalopram.[4] The most common reason for discontinuation was adverse effects; these were reported as the reason for discontinuing the medication by 61%, 57%, and 43% of patients who discontinued the antidepressant at 2, 6, and 12 weeks, respectively.[4] For patients with bipolar disorder taking mood stabilizers, adverse effects are the leading cause of nonadherence to medication.[5] In a survey of patients around the world, 43.5% of respondents reported that at some point in their life, they had discontinued their psychotropic medication due to adverse effects.[6] In clinical trials, the most commonly stated reason for discontinuing antidepressants is adverse events.[7] Thus, the extent to which nonadherence to psychotropic medications is a pervasive problem and seriously hampers the potential utility of treatment needs to be fully appreciated.

ADVERSE EFFECTS ARE CONSIDERED IMPORTANT BY BOTH PATIENTS AND CLINICIANS

In a study using trade-offs, patients considered adverse effects of antidepressants as important as their benefits of symptom relief and relapse prevention.[8] A systematic survey of psychiatrists' prescribing found that the most frequent reason they reported for selecting particular antidepressants was the adverse effects of that antidepressant.[9] Thus, the incidence and nature of adverse effects of an intervention can be a major factor in deciding whether that intervention is considered acceptable and worthwhile.[10] It is, therefore, important to have fairly accurate estimates of the absolute and relative prevalence of various adverse effects with different psychotropic medications.

Table 1
Drug-placebo difference for the most common adverse event of each psychotropic medication

Medication	Adverse Event	Drug-Placebo Difference (%)
Alprazolam	Impaired coordination	22
Aripiprazole (for bipolar mania)	Akathisia	9
Atomoxetine	Nausea	16
Bupropion	Tremor	13.5
Buspirone	Dizziness	9
Citalopram	Ejaculation disorder	5
Clonazepam	Somnolence	27
Clozapine	Drowsiness/sedation	39
Duloxetine	Nausea	15
Escitalopram	Ejaculation disorder	8
Fluoxetine	Nausea	13
Lisdexamfetamine	Decreased appetite	25
Mirtazapine	Somnolence	36
Mixed amphetamine salts	Loss of appetite	30
Modafinil	Nausea	8
Olanzapine	Somnolence	22
Oxcarbazepine	Dizziness	16
Paroxetine (for major depressive disorder)	Nausea	17
Quetiapine (for bipolar depression)	Somnolence	42
Sertraline (for all diagnoses)	Nausea	14
Valproic acid	Nausea	34
Venlafaxine	Nausea	26
Vilazodone (40 mg/d)	Diarrhea	19
Vortioxetine (10 mg/d)	Nausea	17
Zaleplon (5–10 mg/d)	Abdominal pain	3
Ziprasidone (for bipolar mania)	Somnolence	19
Zolpidem	Dizziness	4

Drug-placebo difference for adverse events that occurred at least twice as often on drug as on placebo.

For prescribing clinicians to adequately discuss risks and benefits of medications, they need reliable and complete information about potential adverse effects of medications.[11]

The methodology for evaluating adverse effects of medications is significantly underdeveloped, however, compared with the methodology for assessment of efficacy of medications.[12] Next, I will review some of the problems related to identification and assessment of symptoms and signs that may be adverse effects of the drug.

RATING SCALES FOR ADVERSE EFFECTS ARE INFREQUENTLY USED

Rating scales for adverse effects are not commonly used in clinical trials, except for scales that assess specific objective adverse effects, like extrapyramidal symptoms. For example, only 14% of 73 antidepressant clinical trials used any rating scale for adverse effects, only 18% described assessing the severity of the adverse effects, and only 12% reported assessing persistence of the adverse effects.[13]

CAUSAL ATTRIBUTION IS KEY TO IDENTIFYING ADVERSE EFFECTS

A major problem with how adverse effects were identified and assessed in the clinical trials included in the study discussed previously[13] was that none of the clinical trials included in that study reported using any method to assess the relationship of the adverse events to the study drug, except that the adverse event occurred after starting the study drug.[12] Undesirable events that occur during a clinical trial are noted as adverse events, even if it is very unlikely that there is a causal relationship between the medication and the adverse event.

Clinicians reading the literature on clinical trials need to be aware that in clinical trials, any undesirable problem that a subject encounters, whether related to the drug/placebo or not, is called an adverse event or a treatment-emergent adverse event. The term, adverse effect, on the other hand, generally implies that the undesirable symptom is due to the drug. Clinical trials identify adverse events, not adverse effects.

Only 38%, 44%, and 23%, respectively, of symptoms identified by open-ended questions, a focused interview specific to the medication being used, or a general review of body systems, were attributed to the medication by a physician systematically evaluating a patient for this purpose.[14] Thus, it is important that an assessment be made about how likely it is that the adverse event can be attributed to the medication.

This problem of causal attribution is generally dealt with in one of several ways. In some cases, the investigator is asked to provide a judgment as to whether the adverse event is "possibly related" or "unrelated" to the drug/placebo. There are no guidelines, however, as to the criteria for referring to an adverse event as "possibly related." Also, the term, possible, can be interpreted to include even a remote possibility. For these reasons, referring to some adverse events as "possibly related" to the drug/placebo is considerably subjective. I suspect that given that it is usually difficult to say that the event is "unrelated," an opinion that seems quite definite, in many cases the investigators may be stating instead that it is "possible" that the adverse event is due to the medication. "Possible" may mean "Not impossible".

The other approach to the problem of causal attribution, at least in placebo-controlled clinical trials, is to compare the incidence of each adverse event on drug versus on placebo. The comparison of adverse events on drug versus on placebo, however, is rarely subjected to statistical testing. There are several reasons for this, including that adverse events are not systematically assessed, that a priori hypotheses about adverse events are usually lacking, and that there are numerous comparisons to be made. In any case, lack of statistical significance in comparing the incidence of particular adverse events on drug versus on placebo should not be taken to indicate that there is no difference.[15] This is because due to small sample sizes the possibility of clinically important differences between the groups is not excluded by a statistically nonsignificant result.[16,17]

Because adverse events may occur somewhat more often on drug than on placebo (and vice versa) simply by chance, a common approach is to identify adverse events that occur at least twice as often on drug as on placebo. Although this has intuitive appeal, this approach may exclude some true adverse effects in situations where the incidence of the adverse effect is less than the incidence of the adverse event on placebo. In such situations, the incidence of the adverse event on drug (placebo rate plus adverse effect of the drug) is not at least twice that on placebo.

EXISTING METHODS FOR ASSESSMENT OF ADVERSE EFFECTS HAVE IMPORTANT LIMITATIONS

How patients are assessed for adverse effects significantly affects the frequency of adverse events that are identified.[18] Sometimes investigators or sponsors may change how adverse events are assessed or reported (either the definition of the adverse event or the method of assessment) from commonly used approaches. This may alter the conclusions, eg, the conclusion using an idiosyncratic way of assessing or reporting adverse effects may be that one medication has a better adverse event profile than another.[17]

There are 4 general approaches to identify adverse effects, but each of them has significant limitations.

Spontaneous Reporting by Patients

Clinicians cannot simply rely on patients to spontaneously report any adverse events to them. Of patients who had adverse effects of the antidepressant they were taking, 45.8% reported that they had not discussed these with either their physician or their pharmacist.[1] The reasons why patients do not spontaneously report all adverse events have been little studied. Patients may not realize that certain adverse events may be adverse effects of the medications. Also, patients may be reluctant to report certain adverse events that may be embarrassing (eg, sexual dysfunction).

Open-Ended Questioning

An alternative to waiting for spontaneous reporting is to ask an open-ended question about whether the person has had any new problems or any problems with the medication. This approach, however, often misses symptoms that may be adverse effects. An open-ended question about presence of any adverse effects did not identify 66.7% of adverse effects identified using the combination of a symptom inventory and physician evaluation.[19] Thus, the sensitivity of the open-ended question was only 33.3%. In another study, open-ended questioning identified only 26.8% of adverse effects identified during assessment by a psychiatrist.[20]

It could be argued that if an adverse event is important, the patient will bring it up when asked an open-ended question. In a study using the Systematic Assessment for Treatment-Emergent Events scale, however, of symptoms that led to some medical action (other than simply more careful observation), 46% were not identified on open-ended questioning.[21] Surprisingly, this included 61% of severe adverse events and 65% of events that were causing severe functional impairment. Another finding in this regard has been that management of certain adverse effects significantly improved patients' quality of life even if the patients were not spontaneously complaining about those adverse effects.[22]

Patient-Rated Scales

Examples of patient-rated scales for adverse events include the Patient-Rated Inventory of Side Effects (PRISE)[23]; Frequency, Intensity, and Burden of Side Effects Rating (FIBSER) scale[24]; and a patient-rated version of the UKU Side Effect Rating Scale.[25]

Patient-rated symptom inventories like the PRISE mainly involve asking patients to report the presence or absence of symptoms from a list. A large number of symptoms are often reported; many of these may not be causally related to the medication. In 1 study using a symptom inventory, a mean of 15 symptoms per patient was identified. Only 5.5% of symptoms identified on the symptom inventory were considered by the psychiatrist to be "probable adverse effects" and another 12.5% were considered to be "possible adverse effects."[19]

The FIBSER provides global ratings of the frequency, intensity, and burden of symptoms that a patient considers to side effects but does not identify specific adverse effects (because it was intended to be used along with the PRISE) and the causal attribution is completely subjective. Also, the FIBSER asks patients to "not rate side effects if you believe they are due to treatments that you are taking for medical conditions other than depression," but this is a determination that is probably hard for patients to make.

Clinician-Rated Scales

Examples of clinician-rated scales include the Systematic Assessment for Treatment Emergent Events – General Inquiry and the Systematic Assessment for Treatment Emergent Events – Specific Inquiry,[26] Toronto Side Effect Scale,[27] and the UKU Side Effect Rating Scale.[28]

The clinician-rated scales for adverse effects are time consuming, requiring 30 to 60 minutes to complete.[24,27,29] This discourages their use even in clinical trials. In the case of the Toronto Side Effect Scale, its psychometric properties have not been adequately studied. Also, clinician-rated scales for adverse effects identify symptoms rather than adverse effects because they do not use any standardized method to assess how likely it is that a particular symptom is due to the medication, that is, is really an adverse effect of the medication.[18] This causal attribution is a difficult problem for which the methodology has not been adequately studied.

Thus, these various different methods of identifying adverse effects reviewed fail to identify many adverse effects (ie, have low sensitivity) and identify many symptoms that are probably not adverse effects of the drug (ie, have low positive predictive value).[18]

CHANGES IN VITAL SIGNS AND LABORATORY MEASURES CAN BE ADVERSE EVENTS

Changes in vital signs and in laboratory measures that are considered potentially clinically significant are sometimes specified in clinical trial protocols. This approach is preferable to the common approach of leaving to an investigator's subjective judgment the decision about whether or not to call a change in a vital sign or laboratory test result an adverse event. The same is true of adverse effects identified by use of rating scales for a particular adverse event (eg, tardive dyskinesia or akathisia). In a study evaluating the incidence of tardive dyskinesia, the incidence based on a rating scale for tardive dyskinesia varied from 0% to 5.9% depending on the criteria used, but tardive dyskinesia was identified as a clinical adverse event based on clinical evaluation in only one subject (0.4%).[30]

CLINICAL TRIALS DO NOT ADEQUATELY OR CONSISTENTLY REPORT ADVERSE EFFECTS

Articles reporting the results of clinical trials variously report "the most common adverse events," adverse events that occurred in 5% (or 10%) or more of persons on the drug (or in either group), and so forth. Similarly, in comparing the incidence of adverse events to those on placebo, they report only adverse events that occurred in more persons on drug than on placebo, only those that occurred at least twice as often on drug as on placebo, or use some other criterion.

Clinical decision-making requires information not only on the incidence of each adverse event but also about their severity, persistence, and reversibility. A structured review of articles reporting the results of antidepressant clinical trials found that only 18% of these articles reported on the severity of adverse events, only

12% reported assessing the persistence of adverse events, and only 16% reported what laboratory tests had been done to assess for adverse effects.[12] Poor reporting of data on adverse events is not unique to mental health; it has been found in other specialties as well.[31] A review of product information documents for antidepressants and anticonvulsants also found that these documents listed a large number of adverse events but did not contain contextual information like the duration, severity, and reversibility of those adverse events, information that is important to patients and prescribing clinicians.[10]

For continuous variables, it is unfortunately common to report mean values without describing the percentage of patients who had met a prespecified, clinically meaningful cutoff.[32] Thus, for example, an article may describe that the mean change in weight in patients on the drug was 0.1 kg, leading a clinician-reader to wrongly conclude that the drug is weight neutral. These mean values may obscure the fact that a significant minority of patients had more significant weight gain.

Constraints of word limits often limit how much information about adverse events can be provided in a publication about a clinical trial. Also, due to lack of a standardized approach to reporting adverse events, they were found to be reported inconsistently between the United States and Europe/Australia in the product information for the same medications.[10,33] Similarly, lack of standard terminology is a methodological challenge in being able to adequately summarize data on adverse events into systematic reviews.[34] Attempts to obtain from large systematic reviews meaningful data about adverse events that occur infrequently are hampered because 55.8% of these large systematic reviews did not include data on harms.[16] Since adverse events are poorly reported in clinical trials, the information regarding adverse events that is included in systematic reviews and meta-analyses is inadequate. Such syntheses may even avoid synthesizing or reporting data on adverse events when the available data are of poor quality or highly heterogeneous.[16]

IT IS UNCLEAR HOW EXACTLY TO EDUCATE PATIENTS ABOUT ADVERSE EFFECTS

Good clinical practice and the principles of informed consent suggest that patients should be told about potential adverse effects from the medication that they are about to start. There are few data on how often and how adequately this is done. One challenge is that it is surprisingly hard for clinicians to agree on the precise nature and prevalence of potential adverse effects due to a particular medication, although this does not need to be the case.[35]

One concern sometimes expressed by prescribers is that telling patients about potential adverse effects may cause them to report them more often and potentially discontinue the medication due to these adverse effects. In a study of this issue, patients who reported that they had been informed about potential adverse effects did report mild-to-moderate adverse effects more often but did not prematurely discontinue the medication more often.[3] Also, during the course of treatment, patients who reported discussing adverse effects with their physicians were approximately half as likely to discontinue the antidepressant but more than 5 times as likely to change the antidepressant.[1] This suggests, consistent with clinical observation, that reporting and discussing any adverse effects with the prescribing clinician may lead to the antidepressant being changed, which may help patients to stay on an antidepressant. I am unaware of any data, however, that show that educating patients about potential adverse effects may lead to increased discontinuation of treatment due to adverse effects.

THERE IS LITTLE RESEARCH INTO MANAGEMENT OF ADVERSE EFFECTS

Clinical trials for the prevention and treatment of most adverse events are sparse in the literature. As an example, for the common adverse event of antidepressant-induced excessive sweating, no clinical trial of any treatment had been conducted more than half a century after the introduction of antidepressants. The first clinical trial of any treatment of this persistent and bothersome adverse effect was conducted in 2013.[36] In addition, the clinical trials for management of adverse effects tend to be underpowered.

Given the importance of adverse effects and the many problems related to their assessment and management, what should be done? For the consideration of researchers, clinicians, professional societies, and journal editors, I propose the following plan of action for assessment and reporting of adverse events, educating patients about potential adverse effects, and management of adverse effects.

RECOMMENDATIONS FOR ASSESSMENT OF ADVERSE EFFECTS

Regulatory agencies like the US Food and Drug Administration provide limited specific guidance about how adverse events must be identified or reported. Guidelines for assessment and reporting of adverse events in clinical trials need to be developed and voluntarily adopted. An ideal approach to identification and assessment of adverse effects in clinical trials would include all of the following[18]:

1. Identification of all symptoms that are present while on the drug or placebo
2. Systematic and standardized assessment of the causal relationship between the drug and each symptom
3. Rating of the severity of each adverse effect and functional impairment caused by it, which is relevant to appreciating its clinical significance
4. Repeated administration of the instrument being used to identify and assess adverse effects to allow determination of how long each adverse effect persists and how its severity changes.

The following measures are recommended:

1. A standardized way of asking patients about any adverse events using open-ended questioning should be adopted. Instead of simply using spontaneously reported adverse events, open-ended questioning using specified, standard language should be required at each visit and the subjects' responses noted.
2. In addition to open-ended questions, rating scales to actively screen for any adverse events should be required. Such rating scales should not only identify any adverse events that may have occurred but also assess their severity.
3. A combination of rating scales for adverse events is needed, including scales aimed at identifying and assessing specific adverse effects (eg, akathisia, parkinsonism, and sexual dysfunction) and those that aim to identify a variety of adverse events.
4. New general rating scales that identify and assess a broad variety of adverse effects should be developed and evaluated.[18,19]
5. Standard definitions for the severity of adverse effects should be adopted—across trials, when possible, or for that particular trial if needed.
6. For vital signs, laboratory measures, and adverse events assessed using standardized rating scales (eg, akathisia and tardive dyskinesia), definitions of changes that constitute a potentially clinically significant adverse event should be standardized and prespecified in the protocol rather than leaving the determination to the subjective judgment of the investigator.

7. When investigators are asked to give an opinion about the potential association between the adverse event and the drug, careful attention should be paid to the terminology because it is difficult for an investigator to be certain that an adverse event either is or is not due to the drug. Therefore, using the term, *unlikely to be related*, may be used more often than the term, *unrelated*, although this has not yet been empirically tested.
8. Further research is needed into the problem of causal attribution and the effects of reporting adverse events that occur more often on the drug than on placebo, or twice as often, or statistically significantly more often.

RECOMMENDATIONS FOR REPORTING OF ADVERSE EFFECTS

Although the Consolidated Standards of Reporting Trials (CONSORT) statement guidelines[37] on reporting of randomized clinical trials and their most recent update[9] include only 1 item on reporting adverse events, an extension aiming at better reporting of harms has been published.[15] This extension made a series of recommendations related to the reporting of harms. Some of their recommendations are that a report of a clinical trial should mention the following:

1. If harms were addressed by the study (in the title/abstract and in the introduction)
2. The adverse events assessed by the study, along with their definitions, either standardized, validated ones, or new definitions
3. When appropriate, the severity of the adverse events and whether or not they were unexpected
4. Details of how harms-related information was collected
5. How the data on harms will be presented and analyzed
6. Any subgroup analysis of the data on harms
7. A balanced discussion of benefit and harms

I strongly recommend review of this extension of the CONSORT guidelines.[15] In addition to their recommendations on reporting, I also suggest the following:

1. The criteria for including adverse events in the article should be explicitly specified, preferably in advance.
2. At a minimum, all adverse events that occur in 5% or more of persons on the drug and at least twice as often as on placebo should be reported.
3. In addition to these common adverse events, however, other adverse events that are serious and/or unexpected should be reported.
4. Based on standard definitions, the severity of each adverse effect that occurs should be reported because this information is needed for appreciating the clinical significance of that adverse effect.
5. For each adverse event, the time course of the adverse event should be reported because this information is needed by patients and clinicians to make informed decisions regarding treatment.
6. Because mean changes in variables may not reveal clinically significant changes in a few subjects, reporting of potentially clinically significant changes should be required.
7. Systematic reviews and meta-analyses must also include data on adverse events in addition to those on efficacy. This is particularly important for adverse events that occur infrequently (1% or fewer of subjects) because individual clinical trials may not be adequately powered to provide data on these infrequently occurring adverse events.

8. Online supplements should be used to overcome the problem of space constraints so that full details can be provided about how adverse events were identified and assessed and about the findings.

RECOMMENDATIONS FOR EDUCATING PATIENTS ABOUT ADVERSE EFFECTS

I recommend that, at minimum, patients should be told about

1. All adverse events that occur at least twice as often as on placebo and that occur in at least 5% more patients than on placebo.[33] The rationale for this is (1) that adverse events that occur at least twice as often as on placebo are more likely to be true adverse effects and (2) a drug-placebo difference of 5% means that the undesirable event was probably an adverse event in 5% of subjects.
2. In addition, patients must also be told about potentially serious or life-threatening adverse effects even if they occur infrequently.

Ironically, adverse effects that lead most frequently to discontinuation tend to be ones that are not medically serious. For example, the adverse effects most frequently reported as a reason for discontinuing SSRIs were drowsiness/fatigue, anxiety, headache, and nausea.[3] Thus, patients should be educated that most adverse effects are "nuisance side effects." Although they are bothersome and do need to be managed in some way, patients find it helpful to know that these adverse effects do not indicate that the medication is harming any organ of their body.

If objective criteria are developed for deciding on what should be told to patients, consensus documents can be prepared rather than each clinician developing his or her own education for that medication.

RECOMMENDATIONS REGARDING MANAGEMENT OF ADVERSE EFFECTS

For most adverse effects, the management strategies recommended are based on case reports or clinical experience. Clinical trials for the prevention and treatment of adverse effects that are clinically important need to be given more attention than they currently are. As discussed previously, for antidepressant-induced excessive sweating, a common, distressing, and persistent adverse effect of almost all antidepressants, no clinical trial of any treatment was conducted until recently.[34] Similarly, for drug holidays as a strategy for managing antidepressant-induced sexual dysfunction, an uncontrolled clinical trial published in 1995 was positive,[38] but no confirmatory study has been done since then. For many adverse effects, no clinical trial of any treatment strategy has ever been done.

Adverse effects may be prevented or reduced by different strategies but these need to be empirically tested and widely adopted. For example, nausea due to duloxetine can be reduced by titrating up the medication[39] or by taking it with food.[40]

SUMMARY

Side effects are not a side issue. The most important problem of psychopharmacology is nonadherence and one of the most common causes of nonadherence is adverse effects. Adverse effects also cause patient suffering sometimes equaling and at times even exceeding suffering due to the illness itself. Adverse effects need to be viewed not as a necessary and unavoidable price to be paid for the benefits of treatment but as a major cause of suffering and nonadherence that need to be energetically prevented, reduced, and managed. Clinical researchers and funding agencies need to focus substantial research efforts to develop better approaches to assessment, reporting, and management of adverse effects.

REFERENCES

1. Bull SA, Hu XH, Hunkeler EM, et al. Discontinuation of use and switching of antidepressants: influence of patient-physician communication. JAMA 2002; 288(11):1403–9.
2. Hu XH, Bull SA, Hunkeler EM, et al. Incidence and duration of side effects and those rated as bothersome with selective serotonin reuptake inhibitor treatment for depression: patient report versus physician estimate. J Clin Psychiatry 2004;65(7):959–65.
3. Bull SA, Hunkeler EM, Lee JY, et al. Discontinuing or switching selective serotonin-reuptake inhibitors. Ann Pharmacother 2002;36(4):578–84.
4. Crawford AA, Lewis S, Nutt D, et al. Adverse effects from antidepressant treatment: randomised controlled trial of 601 depressed individuals. Psychopharmacology (Berl) 2014;231(15):2921–31.
5. Mago R, Borra D, Mahajan R. Role of adverse effects in medication nonadherence in bipolar disorder. Harv Rev Psychiatry 2014;22(6):363–6.
6. Wang PS, Gilman SE, Guardino M, et al. Initiation of and adherence to treatment for mental disorders: examination of patient advocate group members in 11 countries. Med Care 2000;38(9):926–36.
7. Roose SP. Compliance: the impact of adverse events and tolerability on the physician's treatment decisions. Eur Neuropsychopharmacol 2003;13(suppl 3): S85–92.
8. Wouters H, Van Dijk L, Van Geffen EC, et al. Primary-care patients' trade-off preferences with regard to antidepressants. Psychol Med 2014;44(11):2301–8.
9. Zimmerman M, Posternak M, Friedman M, et al. Which factors influence psychiatrists' selection of antidepressants? Am J Psychiatry 2004;161:1285–9.
10. Moher D, Hopewell S, Schulz KF, et al, Consolidated Standards of Reporting Trials Group. CONSORT 2010 Explanation and Elaboration: Updated guidelines for reporting parallel group randomised trials. J Clin Epidemiol 2010;63(8):e1–37.
11. Cornelius VR, Liu K, Peacock J, et al. Variation in adverse drug reactions listed in product information for antidepressants and anticonvulsants, between the USA and Europe: a comparison review of paired regulatory documents. BMJ Open 2016;6(3):e010599.
12. Greenhill LL, Vitiello B, Riddle MA, et al. Review of safety assessment methods used in pediatric psychopharmacology. J Am Acad Child Adolesc Psychiatry 2003;42:627–33.
13. Woodmansee C, Mago R, Shah S, et al. Identification and assessment of adverse effects in antidepressant clinical trials. San Diego (CA): American Psychiatric Association; 2007.
14. Greenhill LL, Vitiello B, Fisher P, et al. Comparison of increasingly detailed elicitation methods for the assessment of adverse events in pediatric psychopharmacology. J Am Acad Child Adolesc Psychiatry 2004;43:1488–96.
15. Jonville-Béra AP, Giraudeau B, Autret-Leca E. Reporting of drug tolerance in randomized clinical trials: when data conflict with authors' conclusions. Ann Intern Med 2006;144(4):306–7.
16. Ioannidis JP, Evans SJ, Gøtzsche PC, et al, CONSORT Group. Better reporting of harms in randomized trials: an extension of the CONSORT statement. Ann Intern Med 2004;141(10):781–8.

17. Papanikolaou PN, Ioannidis JP. Availability of large-scale evidence on specific harms from systematic reviews of randomized trials. Am J Med 2004;117(8): 582–9.

18. Ioannidis JP, Mulrow CD, Goodman SN. Adverse events: the more you search, the more you find. Ann Intern Med 2006;144(4):298–300.

19. Mago R, Kloos A, Daskalakis C, et al. Identifying potential adverse effects by patients' ratings: a proof-of-concept study of a novel approach. J Clin Psychopharmacol 2012;32(6):828–31.

20. Mago R, Huhn K, Schwarz M. A Novel Symptom Assessment Tool for Potential Adverse Effects. Poster presented at the 169th annual meeting of the American Psychiatric Association. Atlanta, Georgia, May 14-18, 2016.

21. Levine J, Schooler NR. General versus specific inquiry with SAFTEE. J Clin Psychopharmacol 1992;12:448.

22. Lampela P, Hartikainen S, Sulkava R, et al. Adverse drug effects in elderly people—disparity between clinical examination and adverse effects self-reported by the patient. Eur J Clin Pharmacol 2007;63:509–15.

23. Rush AJ, Fava M, Wisniewski SR, et al, STAR*D Investigators Group. Sequenced treatment alternatives to relieve depression (STAR*D): rationale and design. Control Clin Trials 2004;25(1):119–42.

24. Wisniewski SR, Rush AJ, Balasubramani GK, et al, STARD Investigators. Self-rated global measure of the frequency, intensity, and burden of side effects. J Psychiatr Pract 2006;12(2):71–9.

25. Lindstrom E, Lewander T, Malm U, et al. Patient-rated versus clinician-rated side effects of drug treatment in schizophrenia. Clinical validation of a self-rating version of the UKU Side Effect Rating Scale (UKU-SERS-Pat). Nord J Psychiatry 2001;55(Suppl 44):5–69.

26. Levine J, Schooler NR. SAFTEE: a technique for the systematic assessment of side effects in clinical trials. Psychopharmacol Bull 1986;22(2):343–81.

27. Vanderkooy JD, Kennedy SH, Bagby RM. Antidepressant side effects in depression patients treated in a naturalistic setting: a study of bupropion, moclobemide, paroxetine, sertraline, and venlafaxine. Can J Psychiatry 2002;47(2):174–80.

28. Lingjaerde O, Ahlfors UG, Bech P, et al. The UKU side effect rating scale. A new comprehensive rating scale for psychotropic drugs and a cross-sectional study of side effects in neuroleptic-treated patients. Acta Psychiatr Scand Suppl 1987;334:1–100.

29. Day JC, Wood G, Dewey M, et al. A self-rating scale for measuring neuroleptic side-effects. Validation in a group of schizophrenic patients. Br J Psychiatry 1995;166(5):650–3.

30. Blumberger DM, Mulsant BH, Kanellopoulos D, et al. The incidence of tardive dyskinesia in the study of pharmacotherapy for psychotic depression. J Clin Psychopharmacol 2013;33(3):391–7.

31. Ioannidis JP, Lau J. Completeness of safety reporting in randomized trials: an evaluation of 7 medical areas. JAMA 2001;285:437–43.

32. Mago R, Mahajan R, Thase ME. Medically serious adverse effects of newer antidepressants. Curr Psychiatry Rep 2008;10(3):249–57.

33. Aagaard L, Hansen EH. Adverse drug reaction labelling for atomoxetine, methylphenidate and modafinil: comparison of product information for oral formulations in Australia, Denmark and the United States. Curr Drug Saf 2013;8(3):162–8.

34. Hopewell S, Wolfenden L, Clarke M. Reporting of adverse events in systematic reviews can be improved: survey results. J Clin Epidemiol 2008;61(6):597–602.

35. Mago R. Side effects of psychiatric medications: prevention, assessment, and management. Seattle, WA: Amazon Digital Services, Inc; 2014.
36. Mago R, Thase ME, Rovner BW. Antidepressant-Induced Excessive Sweating: Clinical Features and Treatment with Terazosin. Ann Clin Psychiatry 2013;25(2): E1–7.
37. Altman DG, Schulz KF, Moher D, et al, CONSORT GROUP (Consolidated Standards of Reporting Trials). The revised CONSORT statement for reporting randomized trials: explanation and elaboration. Ann Intern Med 2001;134(8):663–94.
38. Rothschild AJ. Selective serotonin reuptake inhibitor-induced sexual dysfunction: efficacy of a drug holiday. Am J Psychiatry 1995;152(10):1514–6.
39. Dunner DL, Wohlreich MM, Mallinckrodt CH, et al. Clinical consequences of initial duloxetine dosing strategies: comparison of 30 and 60 mg QD starting doses. Curr Ther Res Clin Exp 2005;66(6):522–40.
40. Whitmyer VG, Dunner DL, Kornstein SG, et al. A comparison of initial duloxetine dosing strategies in patients with major depressive disorder. J Clin Psychiatry 2007;68(12):1921–30.

Core Concepts Involving Adverse Psychotropic Drug Effects
Assessment, Implications, and Management

Joseph F. Goldberg, MD[a],*, Carrie L. Ernst, MD[a,b]

KEYWORDS

- Nocebo • Adverse effects • Adverse event • Pharmacogenetics • Iatrogenic
- Drug safety • Drug tolerability

KEY POINTS

- Adverse drug effects occur in more than half of patients taking medications for major psychiatric disorders; but their potential to jeopardize treatment adherence often depends on patient expectations, adverse effect severity, illness severity, alternative pharmacotherapies, and viable ways to manage the adverse effects.
- Patient characteristics that may increase the risk for developing adverse effects include negative treatment expectations, suggestibility, emotionality, proneness to somatization, phobic-obsessive traits, slow metabolizer phenotypes, and historical sensitivity to adverse drug effects.
- Pharmacogenetic markers are beginning to yield useful information about patient-specific vulnerabilities to certain adverse drug effects and overall adverse effect severity.
- A systematic approach to the assessment of suspected adverse drug effects can help optimize therapeutic outcomes.

Adverse effects from psychotropic drugs account for nearly 90,000 annual visits to emergency departments in the United States,[1] yet their management remains among the least studied problems within clinical psychopharmacology. Sheer suspicion about the possible presence of a drug adverse effect brings together concerns

Disclosure: In the past 12 months, J.F. Goldberg has been a consultant to Myriad Genetics, Suno-vion, WebMD, and Medscape. He has served on the speakers' bureau for AstraZeneca, Janssen, Merck, Sunovion, Vanda Pharmaceuticals, and Takeda-Lundbeck. He has received an editorial stipend from Frontline Medical Communications and royalties from American Psychiatric Publishing, Inc., United States. C.L. Ernst has received royalties from American Psychiatric Publishing, Inc., United States.
[a] Department of Psychiatry, Icahn School of Medicine at Mount Sinai, Gustave L. Levy Place, Box 1230, New York, NY 10029, USA; [b] Department of Medical Education, Icahn School of Medicine at Mount Sinai, Gustave L. Levy Place, Box 1230, New York, NY 10029, USA
* Corresponding author. 128 East Avenue, Norwalk, CT 06851.
E-mail address: joseph.goldberg@mssm.edu

regarding pharmacodynamics, pharmacokinetics, pharmacogenetics, psychosomatics, psychodynamics, treatment expectations, drug adherence, and the therapeutic alliance. Because drugs do not differentially exert beneficial versus adverse consequences, it falls to the prescriber to understand fully the end-organ effects of a given medication, alongside the plausibility, time course, dosing relationships, drug interactions, and interplay of pharmacodynamic and psychological factors that collectively become manifest as physical, behavioral, and cognitive-emotional symptoms.

This article reviews basic concepts related to the aforementioned considerations involving the assessment and management of putative adverse effects of psychotropic drugs. The authors first consider the extent to which patient and prescriber expectations about possible adverse effects can influence treatment outcome, alongside patient- and medication-specific factors that seem to moderate the emergence of adverse drug effects.

IMPACT OF ADVERSE EFFECTS ON ADHERENCE: ANTICIPATION VERSUS ACTUAL OCCURRENCE

Rates of nonadherence to psychotropic medications due specifically to adverse effects, or at least the perception of adverse effects, have been reported to range from 14% (in bipolar disorder[2]) to 30% (in schizophrenia[3]). Among depressed older adults who newly begin an antidepressant, adverse effects accounted for about a 5% increase in the probability of treatment discontinuation.[4] Presence of somatic symptoms of depression at baseline may especially predict discontinuation due to adverse effects during antidepressant treatment.[5]

Magnitude and severity of adverse effects also influence outcome; among depressed patients at a 3-month follow-up, incurring one or more rated as being "extremely bothersome" adverse effects increased the chances of antidepressant discontinuation by 150%, but adverse effect presence alone (or less severe adverse effects) did not.[6] Treatment discontinuation due to adverse effects also may correlate with higher doses of selective serotonin reuptake inhibitors (SSRIs).[7] *Initial* adverse effects from SSRIs during depression treatment do not seem to increase the likelihood of premature discontinuation in SSRI clinical trials for major depression.[8]

Although adverse effects are often presumed to contribute prominently to medication refusal or nonadherence, attitudes and expectations about medication effects may actually play a more fundamental role. For example, *fear* of possible adverse effects[9] and general beliefs that medications cause harm[10] are more common among drug-nonadherent than adherent patients who have mood disorders. Negative expectations about drug effects also correlate more strongly with *subjective* than *objective* manifestations of putative adverse effects.[11] In the Texas Medication Algorithm Project, patients' negative beliefs about possible harmfulness of medications significantly predicted discontinuation of treatment at both 6 and 12 months.[12] Another study of antidepressant prescribing in primary care found that fears and concerns about adverse drug effects, but not concerns about illness, significantly predicted nonadherence.[13] In schizophrenia, poor antipsychotic medication adherence has been linked with suspected drug-related adverse effects that are more psychological (eg, poor concentration, anxiety, and fatigue) than somatic.[14]

PREDICTORS OF ADVERSE DRUG EFFECTS

A dilemma arises when deciding how best to counsel patients about the likelihood of an adverse effect without generating greater expectations for their occurrence. On the one hand, more than half of patients with a mood disorder think they are often given inadequate information about psychotropic drug adverse effects[15]; but on the other hand, depressed patients who are told about specific adverse effects may be significantly more likely to experience them.[16] However, evidence is mixed to support the validity of the so-called expectancy hypothesis of adverse drug effects during pharmacotherapy for major depression (ie, that forewarning about an adverse effect increases the chance of its occurrence).[17] Another model, described as the "conditioning hypothesis,"[17] holds that past experience of adverse effects from prior medication trials might increase the probability of recapitulating adverse effects with a new medication, although there is little evidence to support this position.[17]

Clinical wisdom often dictates that practitioners tailor their presentations of possible treatment expectations (both adverse and beneficial) to the patient, according to his or her history and psychology. Especially among those who express substantial concerns about treatment safety, or self-identify as highly sensitive to adverse effects, one might proactively lay groundwork for managing adverse effect expectancy via questions, such as the following:

- *"How much detail would you like to know in advance about possible medication adverse effects?"*
- *"Does the power of suggestion tend to make you worry? If so, we should take that into account when discussing medicine effects, both good and bad."*
- *"If you were to look up information about a medicine and read something about a possible adverse effect that troubled you, do you think you could discuss your concerns with me before changing anything about the treatment plan we come up with together?"*

The impact of actual or anticipated adverse drug effects during long-term psychopharmacotherapy is complex and may vary across diagnoses, age groups, illness severity, perceived efficacy, and organ systems affected. Studies involving various diagnoses reveal that clinicians often rate patients' adverse effects as less frequent and severe than when patients self-rate adverse effects.[18] Poor antidepressant adherence among depressed patients may be influenced more by severity of depression symptoms than by actual adverse drug effects.[19] Surveys of depressed patients identify weight gain, sexual dysfunction, and lethargy as among the most debilitating of actual adverse antidepressant effects, leading directly to nonadherence in about 20% to 30% of patients.[20]

Increased adverse effect burden (severity and/or number), in general, has been reported in connection with several factors, including

- Greater severity of depression[8,17,19,21]
- Late onset of response to antidepressants[22]
- Multiple psychiatric comorbidities[21]
- Higher medication dose[7,21]
- Younger age[21]

Clinical and demographic factors that may confer an increased propensity to develop particular adverse psychotropic drug effects are described in **Table 1**.

DOSE RELATIONSHIPS

Clinicians and patients often assume linear dose relationships exist with drug efficacy as well as with adverse effect severity. In fact, neither is true in all instances. **Table 2** provides a summary of adverse effects of psychotropic agents or drug classes for

Table 1
Clinical and demographic correlates of representative treatment-emergent adverse effects from psychotropic drugs

Adverse Effect	Drug/Class	Reported Findings
Antidepressant-associated activation/agitation	Antidepressants	• Family history of major depression (10-fold risk) or other affective disorder (5-fold risk)[23] • Comorbid personality disorder[24]
Dystonic reactions	First-generation antipychotics	• Higher dose[25,26] • Younger age[26–28] (but less robust predictor of EPS over time[28]) • Greater symptom severity[27] • Negative symptoms[27]
Extrapyramidal symptoms	Antipsychotics	Family history of movement disorders[29] • Duration of exposure[29]
Hyperglycemia/risk for diabetes	Olanzapine	• Higher baseline serum glucose (schizophrenia)[30] • Rapid weight gain[30] • Substantial increase in triglycerides[30]
Hypertension	Desvenlafaxine	Higher baseline blood pressure, greater BMI, higher dose, history of hypertension, older age, male sex[31]
Hypothyroidism	Lithium	Weight gain in first year[32]
Renal insufficiency	Lithium	High dosing; multiple daily dosing[33]
Suicidal ideation	Antidepressants	• Age $\leq$24 y • Comorbid substance abuse[34] • Greater severity of depression/melancholic features[34]
Weight gain	Antidepressants	• Low education level[35] • Low BMI[35] • Family history of obesity[35] • Female sex[21] • Greater duration of use[21] • Weight change in first week[36]
	Antidepressant + atypical antipsychotic	Female sex (treatment of psychotic depression)[37]
	Olanzapine	• Rapid initial increase in BMI (bipolar disorder)[38] • Male sex (schizophrenia)[39]

Abbreviations: BMI, body mass index; EPS, extrapyramidal side effects.

which dose relationships are relatively well established. Less clear, however, is the extent to which dose relationships play a role in such common, vexing adverse effects as iatrogenic weight gain, sedation, and cardiovascular dysfunction. Findings regarding dose relationships in these domains vary across agents, are often not well studied, and can remain subject to conjecture and extrapolation. For example, weight gain seems *not* to be dose related in the case of olanzapine but may be with at least some other atypical antipsychotics. Incident rates of sedation due to antihistamine (H_1) blocking effects of atypical antipsychotics, such as quetiapine, seem to be relatively similar across the range of usual therapeutic doses.[41] There is no definitive consensus on whether antipsychotic- or antidepressant-associated orthostatic hypotension, caused by alpha$_1$ adrenergic blockade, is dose dependent.

Table 2
Known dose relationships involving adverse psychotropic drug effects

Adverse Effect	Agent
Akathisia, dystonic reactions, EPS	Antipsychotics
Ataxia	Anticonvulsants
Blurry vision	Lamotrigine, oxcarbazepine
Complex sleep behaviors	Zolpidem[40]
Diastolic hypertension	Venlafaxine
Headache	Modafinil
Hyperprolactinemia	Antipsychotics
Hypothyroidism	Quetiapine
Nausea	Divalproex, escitalopram, iloperidone, lamotrigine, oxcarbazepine, paroxetine, quetiapine, topiramate, vortioxetine
Paresthesias	Topiramate
QTc prolongation	Antipsychotics, citalopram
Sedation	Mirtazapine (inverse dose relationship)
Seizures	Bupropion, clozapine
Sexual dysfunction	Most serotonergic antidepressants
Sweating	SSRIs, SNRIs
Thrombocytopenia	Divalproex
Yawning	Citalopram

Abbreviations: EPS, extrapyramidal side effects; SNRI, serotonin-norepinephrine reuptake inhibitor.
Adapted from Goldberg JF, Ernst CL. Managing the side effects of psychotropic medications. Washington, DC: American Psychiatric Publishing, Inc; 2012. p. 30.

The scant literature in this area includes evidence both for[42] and against[43] such a relationship.

To summarize, clinicians should not automatically assume that all adverse effects follow linear dose relationships or that dosage reductions will routinely ameliorate or reverse their impact. Practically speaking, it is often nevertheless reasonable to reduce a medication dosage in order to determine empirically if an adverse effect may diminish, provided that therapeutic benefits are not sacrificed.

NOCEBO EFFECTS

Adverse effects while taking a pharmacodynamically inert substance pose an intriguing, poorly understood phenomenon. In randomized clinical trials of pharmacotherapy for major depression, common adverse effects associated with placebo (as reported in >10% of subjects) include dizziness, headache, nausea, diarrhea, sedation, insomnia, anorexia, nervousness, and anxiety (Goldberg and Ernst[41[pp18]]). Half or more of placebo-treated patients with major depression experience at least one adverse event, and about 5% prematurely discontinue study participation because of perceived adverse effects while taking placebo.[17,44] Psychological constructs, such as suggestibility, emotionality, and phobic-obsessive traits,[45] have all been linked with a greater likelihood of adverse effects during pharmacotherapy trials for adults with mood or anxiety disorders.

ADVERSE EFFECTS VERSUS NATURAL COURSE OF ILLNESS

It can be particularly challenging to differentiate suspected iatrogenic effects from the persistence or worsening of symptoms of the primary illness. Psychiatric symptoms, such as anxiety, suicidal thinking or behavior, agitation, psychosis, mania, or depression, are all identified as possible adverse effects of many psychotropic agents, yet it often becomes a matter of debate whether a worsening of psychiatric symptoms occurs *because of* or *despite* a given treatment. Paradoxic drug effects over time, such as iatrogenic worsening of depression in patients who are unipolar depressed, termed the "oppositional model of tolerance," which posits that long-term treatment with some drugs may recruit physiologic processes that ultimately oppose their initial acute effects.[46] Strategies to help minimize confusion about cause and effect include

- Making only gradual medication/dosing changes
- Changing only one medication at a time
- Using symptom rating scales to minimize subjectivity about worsening
- Considering at-risk groups (eg, suicidality in antidepressant recipients <24 years of age)
- Obtaining corroborative information from a trusted collateral historian
- Recognizing other features within a symptom constellation that suggest disease progression rather than isolated iatrogenic phenomena

TIME COURSE

As much as one tries to anticipate *when* a drug's therapeutic benefits are most likely to occur, so too can the adverse effects of a drug often emerge along a more or less predictable time course, further helping to corroborate a causal relationship between a particular medication and a putative adverse effect. Knowledge about such temporal relationships can also help forecast expectations about an adverse effect's eventual resolution versus persistence. Examples of adverse effects that typically arise early versus later in the course of medication use are summarized in **Table 3**.

When a clinician forecasts transient adverse effects that usually resolve promptly (with conservative interventions, if any), distress is minimized and trust in the

Table 3	
Time course to emergence of adverse effects	
Early	**Late**
Allergic reactions	Diabetes or hypercholesterolemia from atypical antipsychotics
Extrapyramidal effects	
Hypersensitivity reactions	Tardive dyskinesia from antipsychotics
Cutaneous reactions from lamotrigine (first 2–8 wk)	Weight gain from antidepressants, lithium, divalproex (as contrasted with a swifter time course with many atypical antipsychotics[47])
Myocarditis from clozapine (first 4–8 wk)	
Agranulocytosis from clozapine (highest risk in first 18 wk of treatment)	Renal insufficiency from lithium (in absence of overdose/toxicity; risk for lithium-associated renal insufficiency due solely to long-term use remains in dispute[48])
Neuroleptic malignant syndrome (two-thirds of cases arise within 1 wk of starting an antipsychotic)	
Sedation	Bone demineralization from carbamazepine or SSRIs

Abbreviation: SSRI, selective serotonin reuptake inhibitor.

therapeutic alliance is likely enhanced. Nausea and headache, for example, are common early adverse effects from SSRIs that typically resolve spontaneously within 1 to 2 weeks after initiation. More difficult are adverse effects that tend to persist with a lower likelihood of spontaneously resolving over time, such as anticholinergic effects (eg, dry mouth, constipation),[49] antidepressant-associated sexual dysfunction, excessive sweating,[49] and weight gain. Somnolence from H_1 antagonism is often touted as a strategy to treat chronic insomnia without tolerance, but that attribute also suggests a low likelihood of habituation to antihistaminergic sedation when undesired. Antidepressant-associated sexual dysfunction seems to be dose related with most agents with the notable exceptions of fluoxetine and mirtazapine,[50] and tolerance seems to develop in less than 10% of patients over about a 4- to 6-month period.[51–53]

Weight gain associated with many atypical antipsychotics follows a trajectory that tends to eventually plateau (eg, after about 36 weeks in trials of olanzapine for schizophrenia[54] or 52 weeks with olanzapine plus fluoxetine for major depression[55]). *Overall* adverse effect burden with most psychotropics also generally attenuates over time.[21] During SSRI treatment of major depression, Demyttenaere and colleagues[8] found that habituation to adverse effects in general occurred significantly faster in men than women, particularly among recurrent versus first-episode depressed patients.

ADVERSE EFFECT VARIABILITY ACROSS DIAGNOSES

Adverse effects from a particular drug may also vary across different diagnostic groups. This variation becomes especially relevant when drugs also used elsewhere in medicine (such as anticonvulsants in epilepsy) demonstrate adverse effects (eg, cognitive impairment, menstrual irregularities, osteoporosis) that may not necessarily extrapolate neatly to psychiatric populations. For example, incident rates of polycystic ovary syndrome associated with use of divalproex may be higher in women with epilepsy than bipolar disorder.[56] The Food and Drug Administration's registration trials of fluoxetine showed substantially higher rates of nausea or insomnia when used in patients with obsessive-compulsive disorder (OCD) or bulimia than with panic disorder. Incident rates of nocebo effects also vary across mood and anxiety disorder diagnoses; for example, dry mouth, nausea, and somnolence have been reported more often during placebo treatment of chronic depression than acute major depression (Goldberg and Ernst[41(pp18)]).

PHARMACOGENETICS AND ADVERSE EFFECTS

The increasing popularity of commercially available genotyping kits has prompted many clinicians and patients to rely on pharmacogenetic testing to inform (if not guide) decision-making about psychotropic drug prescribing. Although genotyping of known functional single nucleotide polymorphisms (SNPs) is still not well established as a valid means to predict the efficacy of most psychotropic drugs, associations with apparent adverse drug effects have been reported with several identified SNPs involving drug pharmacokinetics, particularly with respect to slow metabolizer phenotypes and cytochrome P450 isoenzyme genotypes, as summarized in **Table 4**. Notably, the slow metabolizer CYP450 2D6 genotype is sufficiently rare (only 6%–10% of whites, 0%–2% of Asians, and 2%–7% of African Americans or Hispanics [Goldberg and Ernst[41(pp68)]]) that it would seem unlikely to account for most patients who present with drug intolerance. Nevertheless, Mago and colleagues[57] observed that among patients with major depression or generalized anxiety disorder, those with (vs without) severe adverse drug effects were significantly more likely to be poor metabolizers at relevant cytochrome P450 enzyme loci.

Table 4
Examples of known pharmacogenetic variants potentially associated with adverse psychotropic drug effects

Suspected Adverse Effect	Causal Drug	Reported Genotypic Variants
Antidepressant-induced mania	SSRIs	5HTT-LPR (SLC6A4 s allele)[58]
Common adverse effects at low doses	All P450 2D6 substrates	CYP450 2D6 (slow metabolizer genotype for drugs that are P450 2D6 substrates)
Extrapyramidal adverse effects	Antipsychotics	• 5HT2 (Cys23Ser variant)[59] • DRD2 (A1 variant of the Taq1A polymorphism)[60] • rs1130214 (AKT1), rs456998 (FCHSD1), rs7211818 (Raptor), and rs1053639 (DDIT4) (4-way interaction of mTOR genes)[61]
	SSRIs	DRD2 (A1 variant of the Taq1A polymorphism)[62]
Hyperprolactinemia	Antipsychotics	DRD2*A1[63]
Nausea	Paroxetine	HTR3B (Tyr129Ser gene)[64]
Sexual dysfunction	SSRIs	GRIA1 (rs 1994862), GRIA3, GRIK2[65,66]
Sialorrhea	Clozapine	DRD4[67]
Stevens Johnson syndrome	Carbamazepine	HLA-B*1502
Antidepressant-associated suicidality	Antidepressants	• TPH 2 (tryptophan hydroxylase 2) rs1386494 (C/T) polymorphism[68] • BDNF rs962369 polymorphism[69]
Weight gain	Antipsychotics	−5HT2C (−759 C/T variant),[70] MC4R, leptin promoter gene variants,[71] 5HTTLPR s/s or s/l genotype[72]

Abbreviations: 5HTT-LPT, serotonin transporter gene linked polymorphic region; 5HT2, serotonin 2 receptor gene; AKT1, serine/threonine-specific protein kinase; BDNF, brain-derived neurotrophic factor; DDIT4, DNA-damage-inducible transcript 4; DRD2, dopamine receptor D2; DRD4, dopamine receptor D4; FCHSD1, SH3 type formin-binding protein gene; GRIA1, glutamate ionotropic receptor AMPA type subunit 1; GRIK2, glutamate ionotropic receptor kainate type subunit 2; GRIA3, glutamate ionotropic receptor AMPA type subunit 3; HLA, human leukocyte antigen; HTR3B, 5-hydroxytryptamine receptor 3B; MC4R, melanocortin 4 receptor; mTOR, mammalian target of rapamycin; TPH2, tryptophan hydroxylase 2.

Because different drugs are often metabolized by different catabolic pathways, or may in some instances be substrates for multiple metabolic routes, universal generalizations about slow metabolism as a genetic explanation may not apply to all patients who report being highly sensitive to adverse effects.

Metabolic phenotypes also can change over time; for example, Preskorn and colleagues[73] showed that 1 in 4 patients with normal variant CYP450 2D6 genotypes can phenoconvert to a slow metabolizer phenotype. Candidate genes that encode pharmacologically relevant proteins (eg, receptors, transporters, or rate-limiting synthetic enzymes) also have not consistently revealed pharmacogenetic associations with adverse effect burden. For example, despite preliminary findings linking certain DRD2 dopamine gene SNPs with antipsychotic-associated extrapyramidal adverse effects (see **Table 4**), more negative than positive findings have been reported examining variants of D1 and D2 dopamine receptor candidate genes.[74–76] Because numerous factors other than possible genetic predispositions influence pharmacodynamic drug effects, it is difficult to know how much and when to apportion genetic explanations for adverse pharmacodynamic effects.

Global adverse effect burden during SSRI (escitalopram) or serotonin norepinephrine reuptake inhibitor (venlafaxine) treatment of major depression recently has been linked with the rs10245483 variant of the ABCB1 gene that encodes p-glycoprotein (which, in turn, regulates brain concentrations of some antidepressants).[77] Additionally, a functional SNP of the 5HT2C gene (rs6644093) has been associated with presumptive serotonergic adverse effects, such as insomnia, gastrointestinal problems, and sexual dysfunction.[78] Reported findings from representative candidate gene studies involving associations with specific adverse drug effects are described in **Table 4**.

DO ADVERSE EFFECTS INFLUENCE DRUG EFFICACY?

Although adverse effects are usually undesired outcomes relative to intended treatment benefits, at least in some instances, drug efficacy has been hypothesized to be linked with untoward effects. Notably, dissociative adverse effects seem to predict robust and sustained antidepressant effects of intravenous ketamine.[79] Weight gain observed during treatment with either olanzapine or placebo correlates with symptom improvement in schizophrenia.[80] In industry-sponsored multicenter trials for OCD, early complaints of anticholinergic effects (eg, dry mouth, constipation) and dizziness increased the likelihood of subsequent favorable response to clomipramine, as did initial sexual dysfunction and nervousness for both clomipramine and fluoxetine.[81] Obviously, these and other adverse effects that may correlate with drug efficacy (eg, thirst with lithium, weight gain with olanzapine, extrapyramidal effects of antipsychotics) could be artifactual (eg, proxies for adherence, time on drug, or dose) or signs of improvement (eg, restoration of lost appetite in depression), potentially obscuring the distinction between a correlate versus predictor of response.

RISK-BENEFIT ANALYSES

Deciding whether or not to discontinue a medication when suspected adverse effects occur depends on thoughtful consideration of many factors, including

- Illness severity and level of disability
- Disruptiveness of adverse effect to patients
- Natural course of a particular adverse effect (ie, likelihood for resolution or worsening)
- Magnitude of improvement and efficacy from current therapy
- Viable alternative treatment options
- Past treatment outcomes
- Availability of pharmacologic or other strategies to counteract adverse effects

When morbidity from a psychiatric disorder is substantial, medications that exert large and clinically meaningful effects usually warrant greater efforts to manage non–life-threatening adverse effects, especially if few comparable alternatives exist (eg, clozapine in schizophrenia; lithium for some patients with bipolar disorder). At the same time, if a drug's efficacy fades or is known to attenuate beyond a certain time frame, there may no longer be justification for incurring further adverse effects. For example, after a bipolar manic episode is stabilized with lithium or divalproex plus an atypical antipsychotic, combination therapy seems beneficial for up to 24 weeks; but beyond that time frame the fairly modest added protection against recurrence seems to become outweighed by the likelihood of ongoing adverse effects (particularly weight gain).[82]

Table 5 The approach to adverse drug event assessment	
Concept	**Considerations for Clinical Decision-Making**
Pharmacodynamic plausibility	Does the suspected adverse effect make sense pharmacodynamically? In patients receiving complex combination drug regimens, what was the most recent change made? Attempt to change only one variable (medication/dose) at a time.
Pharmacokinetics	Consider whether any drug-drug interactions could account for a change in the bioavailability or toxicity of a given agent.
Individual risk and propensities	Has this patient previously experienced similar adverse effects with other medications? Are there recognizable patient-specific characteristics that increase the likelihood a particular adverse effect will occur?
Timing	When did the suspected adverse effect arise relative to start (or most recent dosage change) of the medication?
Severity and seriousness	Differentiate suspected adverse effects that are medically hazardous or potentially life threatening from those that pose only a nuisance.
Disruptiveness	How disruptive or tolerable is a suspected adverse effect to a given patient?
Transience	Is a tolerable suspected adverse effect likely to dissipate spontaneously with time?
Alternative therapy options	Are there alternative agents with comparable efficacy but lesser risk of a particular adverse effect?
Patient preferences	Invite patients to share in medical decision-making by expressing a preference. Do they place greater importance on controlling particular psychiatric symptoms or avoiding a potential adverse effect?
Risk-benefit considerations	Does a unique therapeutic effect or large effect warrant pursuit of strategies to counteract an adverse effect?
Viable antidotes	Pharmacologic antidotes may create their own adverse effects. Do safe and viable antidote strategies exist?

A SYSTEMATIC APPROACH TO EVALUATING SUSPECTED ADVERSE PSYCHOTROPIC DRUG EFFECTS

Thoughtful management of adverse effects involves integrating the foregoing concepts in order to provide optimal psychiatric treatment tailored to the needs of an individual patient. **Table 5** presents a summary of key considerations to assess, minimize, and counteract potential adverse psychotropic drug effects.

SUMMARY

Psychopharmacologic expertise involves recognizing and managing both the beneficial and adverse pharmacodynamic and pharmacokinetic effects of psychotropic medications. Tailoring the best treatment regimen for an individual patient often requires a careful assessment of a drug's relative risks versus benefits. Such an analysis requires differentiating putative adverse effects from illness symptoms, understanding how time course and dosing factors influence negative drug effects, considering pharmacokinetic interactions and pharmacogenetic contributors to drug metabolism, appreciating the psychological dimensions that often mediate patients' expectations about both beneficial and adverse drug effects, distinguishing medically benign from serious adverse effects, and understanding the evidence base and rationale for pursuing pharmacologic strategies to manage adverse drug effects both safely and effectively.

REFERENCES

1. Hampton LM, Daubresse M, Chang HY, et al. Emergency department visits by adults for psychiatric medication adverse effects. JAMA Psychiatry 2014;71: 1006–14.
2. Cooper C, Bebbington P, King M, et al. Why people do not take their psychotropic drugs as prescribed: results of the 2000 National Psychiatric Morbidity Survey. Acta Psychiatr Scand 2007;116:47–53.
3. Lieberman JA, Stroup TS, McEvoy JP, et al. Effectiveness of antipsychotic drugs in patients with chronic schizophrenia. N Engl J Med 2005;353:1209–33.
4. Mark TL, Joish VN, Hay JW, et al. Antidepressant use in geriatric populations: the burden of side effects and interactions and their impact on adherence and costs. Am J Geriatr Psychiatry 2011;19:211–21.
5. Agosti V, Quitkin FM, Stewart JW, et al. Somatization as a predictor of medication discontinuation due to adverse effects. Int Clin Psychopharmacol 2002;17:311–4.
6. Goethe JW, Wooley SB, Cardoni AA, et al. Selective serotonin reuptake inhibitor discontinuation: side effects and other factors that influence medication adherence. J Clin Psychopharmacol 2007;27:451–8.
7. Jakubovski E, Varigonda AL, Freemantle N, et al. Systematic review and meta-analysis: dose response relationship of selective serotonin reuptake inhibitors in major depressive disorder. Am J Psychiatry 2016;173(2):174–83.
8. Demyttenaere K, Albert A, Mesters P, et al. What happens with adverse events during 6 months of treatment with selective serotonin reuptake inhibitors? J Clin Psychiatry 2005;66:859–63.
9. Scott J, Pope M. Nonadherence with mood stabilizers: prevalence and predictors. J Clin Psychiatry 2002;63:384–90.
10. Fawzi W, Abdel Mohsen MY, Hashem AH, et al. Beliefs about medications predict adherence to antidepressants in older adults. Int Psychogeriatr 2012;24:159–69.
11. Kleindienst N, Greil W. Are illness concepts a powerful predictor of adherence to prophylactic treatment in bipolar disorder? J Clin Psychiatry 2004;65:966–74.
12. Warden D, Rush AJ, Carmody TJ, et al. Predictors of attrition during one year of depression treatment: a roadmap to personalized intervention. J Psychiatr Pract 2009;15:113–24.
13. Hunot VM, Horne R, Leese MN, et al. A cohort study of adherence to antidepressants in primary care: the influence of antidepressant concerns and treatment preferences. Prim Care Companion J Clin Psychiatry 2007;9:91–9.
14. Rettenbacher MA, Hofer A, Eder U, et al. Compliance in schizophrenia: psychopathology, side effects, and patients' attitudes toward the illness and medication. J Clin Psychiatry 2004;65:1211–8.
15. Bowskill R, Clatworthy J, Parham R, et al. Patients' perceptions of information received about medication prescribed for bipolar disorder: implications for informed choice. J Affect Disord 2007;100:253–7.
16. Bull SA, Hunkeler EM, Lee JY, et al. Discontinuing or switching selective serotonin- reuptake inhibitors. Ann Pharmacother 2002;36:578–84.
17. Dodd S, Schacht A, Klein K, et al. Nocebo effects in the treatment of major depression: results from an individual study participant-level meta-analysis of the placebo arm of duloxetine clinical trials. J Clin Psychiatry 2015;76:702–11.

18. Lindström E, Lewander T, Malm U, et al. Patient-rated versus clinician-rated side effects of drug treatment in schizophrenia. Clinical validation of a self-rating version of the UKU Side Effect Rating Scale (UKU-SERS-Pat). Nord J Psychiatry 2001;55(Suppl 4):5–69.

19. De las Cuevas C, Peñate W, Sanz EJ. Risk factors for nonadherence to antidepressant to antidepressant treatment in patients with mood disorders. Eur J Clin Pharmacol 2014;70:89–98.

20. Ashton AK, Jamerson BD, L Weinstein BW, et al. Antidepressant-related adverse effects impacting treatment compliance: results of a patient survey. Curr Ther Res Clin Exp 2005;66:96–106.

21. Bet PM, Hugtenburg JG, Penninx BW, et al. Side effects of antidepressants during long-term use in a naturalistic setting. Eur Neuropsychopharmacol 2013;23: 1443–51.

22. Fabbri C, Marsano A, Balestri M, et al. Clinical features and drug induced side effects in early versus late antidepressant responders. J Psychiatr Res 2013; 47:1309–18.

23. Harada T, Inada K, Yamada K, et al. A prospective naturalistic study of antidepressant- induced jitteriness/anxiety syndrome. Neuropsychiatr Dis Treat 2014; 10:2115–21.

24. Harada T, Sakamoto K, Ishigooka J. Incidence and predictors of activation syndrome induced by antidepressants. Depress Anxiety 2008;25:1014–9.

25. Levinson DF, Simpson GM, Singh H, et al. Fluphenazine dose, clinical response, and extrapyramidal symptoms during acute treatment. Arch Gen Psychiatry 1990;47:761–8.

26. Singh H, Levinson DF, Simpson GM, et al. Acute dystonia during fixed-dose neuroleptic treatment. J Clin Pharmacol 1990;10:389–96.

27. Aguilar EJ, Keshavan MS, Martínez-Quiles MD, et al. Predictors of acute dystonia in first-episode psychotic patients. Am J Psychiatry 1994;151:1819–21.

28. Giegling I, Drago A, Schäfer M, et al. Sociodemographic and treatment related variables are poor predictors of haloperidol induced motor side effects. Prog Neuropsychopharmacol Biol Psychiatry 2011;35:74–7.

29. Lencer R, Eismann G, Kasten M, et al. Family history of primary movement disorders as a predictor for neuroleptic-induced extrapyramidal symptoms. Br J Psychiatry 2004;185:465–71.

30. Reaven GM, Lieberman JA, Sethuraman G, et al. In search of moderators and mediators of hyperglycemia with atypical antipsychotic treatment. J Psychiatr Res 2009;43:997–1002.

31. Thase ME, Fayyad R, Cheng RF, et al. Effects of desvenlafaxine on blood pressure in patients treated for major depressive disorder: a pooled analysis. Curr Med Res Opin 2015;31:809–20.

32. Henry C. Lithium side-effects and predictors of hypothyroidism in patients with bipolar disorder: sex differences. J Psychiatry Neurosci 2002;27:104–7.

33. Castro VM, Roberson AM, McCoy TH, et al. Stratifying risk for renal insufficiency among lithium-treated patients: an electronic health record study. Neuropsychopharmacology 2016;41(4):1138–43.

34. Zisook S, Trivedi MH, Warden D, et al. Clinical correlates of the worsening or emergence of suicidal ideation during SSRI treatment of depression: an examination of citalopram in the STAR*D study. J Affect Disord 2009;117(1–2):63–73.

35. Uquz F, Sahingoz M, Gungor B, et al. Weight gain and associated factors in patients using newer antidepressant drugs. Gen Hosp Psychiatry 2015;37:46–8.

36. Himmerich H, Schuld A, Haack M, et al. Early prediction of changes in weight during six weeks of treatment with antidepressants. J Psychiatr Res 2004;38: 485–90.
37. Deligiannidis KM, Rothschild AJ, Barton BA, et al. A gender analysis of the study of pharmacotherapy of psychotic depression (STOP-PD): gender and age as predictors of response and treatment-associated changes in body mass index and metabolic measures. J Clin Psychiatry 2013;74:1003–9.
38. Hennen J, Perlis RH, Sachs G, et al. Weight gain during treatment of bipolar I patients with olanzapine. J Clin Psychiatry 2004;65:1679–87.
39. Basson BR, Kinon BJ, Taylor CC, et al. Factors influencing acute weight change in patients with schizophrenia treated with olanzapine, haloperidol, or risperidone. J Clin Psychiatry 2001;62:231–8.
40. Hwang TJ, Ni HC, Chen HC, et al. Risk predictors for hypnosedative-related complex sleep behaviors: a retrospective, cross-sectional pilot study. J Clin Psychiatry 2010;71:1331–5.
41. Goldberg JF, Ernst CL. Managing the side effects of psychotropic medications. Washington, DC: American Psychiatric Publishing, Inc; 2012.
42. Jana AK, Praharaj SK, Roy N. Olanzapine-induced orthostatic hypotension. Clin Psychopharmacol Neurosci 2015;13:113–4.
43. Silver H, Kogan H, Zlotogorski D. Postural hypotension in chronically medicated schizophrenics. J Clin Psychiatry 1990;51:459–62.
44. Mitsikostas DD, Mantonakis L, Chalarakis N. Nocebo in clinical trials for depression: a meta-analysis. Psychiatry Res 2014;215:82–6.
45. Downing RW, Rickels K, Rickels LA, et al. Nonspecific factors and side effect complaints. Factors affecting the incidence of drowsiness in drug and placebo treated anxious and depressed outpatients. Acta Psychiatr Scand 1979;60: 438–48.
46. Fava GA. Can long-term treatment with antidepressant drugs worsen the course of depression? J Clin Psychiatry 2003;64:123–33.
47. Tohen M, Ketter TA, Zarate CA, et al. Olanzapine versus divalproex sodium for the treatment of acute mania and maintenance of remission: a 47-week study. Am J Psychiatry 2003;160:1263–71.
48. Clos S, Rauchhaus P, Severn A, et al. Long-term effect of lithium maintenance therapy on estimated glomerular filtration rate in patients with affective disorders: a population- based cohort study. Lancet Psychiatry 2015;2(12):1075–83.
49. Mavissakalian MR, Perel JM. The side effect burden of extended imipramine treatment of panic disorder. J Clin Psychopharmacol 2000;20:547–55.
50. Clayton AH, Pradko JF, Croft HA, et al. Prevalence of sexual dysfunction among newer antidepressants. J Clin Psychiatry 2002;63:357–66.
51. Montejo AL, Llorca G, Izquierdo JA, et al. Incidence of sexual dysfunction associated with antidepressant agents: a prospective multicenter study of 1022 outpatients. J Clin Psychiatry 2001;62:10–21.
52. Montejo-González AL, Llorca G, Izquierdo JA, et al. SSRI-induced sexual dysfunction: fluoxetine, paroxetine, sertraline, and fluvoxamine in a prospective, multicenter, and descriptive clinical study of 344 patients. J Sex Marital Ther 1997;23:176–94.
53. Ashton AK, Rosen RC. Accommodation to serotonin reuptake inhibitor-induced sexual dysfunction. J Sex Marital Ther 1998;24(3):191–2.
54. Kinon BJ, Basson BR, Gilmore JA, et al. Long-term olanzapine treatment: weight change and weight-related health factors in schizophrenia. J Clin Psychiatry 2001;62:92–100.

55. Andersen SW, Clemow DB, Corya SA. Long-term weight gain in patients treated with open-label olanzapine in combination with fluoxetine for major depressive disorder. J Clin Psychiatry 2005;66:1468–76.
56. Ernst CL, Goldberg JF. The reproductive safety profile of mood stabilizers, atypical antipsychotics, and broad-spectrum psychotropics. J Clin Psychiatry 2002; 63(suppl 4):42–55.
57. Mago R, Gupta S, Huhn K, et al. Genetic polymorphisms and antidepressant adverse effects or nonresponse. Poster presented at the annual meeting of the American Psychiatric Association. Toronto, Ontario, Canada, May 16–20, 2015.
58. Daray FM, Thommi SB, Ghaemi SN. The pharmacogenetics of antidepressant-induced mania: a systematic review and meta-analysis. Bipolar Disord 2010; 12:702–6.
59. Gunes A, Dahl ML, Spina E, et al. Further evidence for the association between 5-HT2C receptor gene polymorphisms and extrapyramidal side effects in male schizophrenics. Eur J Clin Pharmacol 2008;64:477–82.
60. Güzey C, Scordo MG, Spina E, et al. Antipsychotic-induced extrapyramidal symptoms in patients with schizophrenia: associations with dopamine and serotonin receptor and transporter polymorphisms. Eur J Clin Pharmacol 2007;63: 233–41.
61. Mas S, Gassó P, Ritter MA, et al. Pharmacogenetic predictor of extrapyramidal symptoms induced by antipsychotics: multilocus interaction in the mTOR pathway. Eur Neuropsychopharmacol 2015;25:51–9.
62. Hedenmalm K, Güzey C, Dahl ML, et al. Risk factors for extrapyramidal symptoms during treatment with selective serotonin reuptake inhibitors, including cytochrome P-450 enzyme, and serotonin and dopamine transporter and receptor polymorphisms. J Clin Psychopharmacol 2006;26:192–7.
63. Young RM, Lawford BR, Barnes M, et al. Prolactin levels in antipsychotic treatment of patients with schizophrenia carrying the DRD2*A1 allele. Br J Psychiatry 2004;185:147–51.
64. Sugai T, Suzuki Y, Sawamura K, et al. The effect of 5-hydroxytryptamine 3A and 3B receptor genes on nausea induced by paroxetine. Pharmacogenomics J 2006;6:351–6.
65. Bishop JR, Chae SS, Patel S, et al. Pharmacogenetics of glutamate system genes an SSRI- associated sexual dysfunction. Psychiatry Res 2012;199:74–6.
66. Perlis RH, Laje G, Smoller JW, et al. Genetic and clinical predictors of sexual dysfunction in citalopram-treated depressed patients. Neuropsychopharmacol 2009;34:1819–28.
67. Rajagopal V, Sundaresan L, Rajkumar AP, et al. Genetic association between the DRD4 promoter polymorphism and clozapine-induced sialorrhea. Psychiatr Genet 2014;24:273–6.
68. Musil R, Zill P, Seemüller F, et al. Genetics of emergent suicidality during antidepressive treatment–data from a naturalistic study on a large sample of inpatients with a major depressive episode. Eur Neuropsychopharmacol 2013;23:663–74.
69. Perroud N, Aitchison KJ, Uher R, et al. Genetic predictors of increase in suicidal ideation during antidepressant treatment in the GENDEP project. Neuropsychopharmacology 2009;34:2517–28.
70. Templeman LA, Reynolds GP, Arranz B, et al. Polymorphisms of the 5-HT2C receptor and leptin genes are associated with antipsychotic drug-induced weight gain in Caucasian subjects with a first-episode psychosis. Pharmacogenet Genomics 2005;15:195–200.

71. Kao AC, Müller DJ. Genetics of antipsychotic-induced weight gain: update and current perspectives. Pharmacogenomics 2013;14:2067–83.
72. Smits K, Smits L, Peeters F, et al. Serotonin transporter polymorphisms and the occurrence of adverse events during treatment with selective serotonin reuptake inhibitors. Int Clin Psychopharmacol 2007;22:137–43.
73. Preskorn SH, Kane CP, Lobello K, et al. Cytochrome P450 2D6 phenoconversion is common in patients being treated for depression: implications for personalized medicine. J Clin Psychiatry 2013;74:614–21.
74. Kaiser R, Tremblay PB, Klufmöller F, et al. Relationship between adverse effects of antipsychotic treatment and dopamine D(2) receptor polymorphisms in patients with schizophrenia. Mol Psychiatry 2002;7:695–705.
75. Dolzan V, Plesnicar BK, Serretti A, et al. Polymorphisms in dopamine receptor DRD1 and DRD2 genes and psychopathological and extrapyramidal symptoms in patients on long-term antipsychotic treatment. Am J Med Genet B Neuropsychiatr Genet 2007;144B:809–15.
76. Wu SN, Gao R, Xing HQ, et al. Association of DRD2 polymorphisms and chlorpromazine-induced extrapyramidal syndrome in Chinese schizophrenic patients. Acta Pharmacol Sin 2006;27:966–70.
77. Schatzberg AF, DeBattista C, Lazzeroni LC, et al. ABCB1 genetic effects on antidepressant response: a report from the iSPOT-D trial. Am J Psychiatry 2015;172:751–9.
78. Hodgson H, Uher R, Crawford AA, et al. Genetic predictors of antidepressant side effects: a grouped candidate gene approach in the Genome-Based Therapeutic Drugs for Depression (GENDEP) study. J Psychopharmacol 2014;28:142–50.
79. Luckenbaugh DA, Niciu MJ, Iosifescu DF, et al. Do the dissociative side effects of ketamine mediate its antidepressant effects. J Affect Disord 2014;159:56–61.
80. Ascher-Svanum H, Stensland MD, Kinon BJ, et al. Weight gain as a prognostic indicator of therapeutic improvement during acute treatment of schizophrenia with placebo or active antipsychotic. J Psychopharmacol 2005;19(6 Suppl):110–7.
81. Ackerman DL, Greenland S, Bystritsky A. Side effects as predictors of drug response in obsessive-compulsive disorder. J Clin Psychopharmacol 1999;19:459–65.
82. Yatham LN, Beaulieu S, Schaffer A, et al. Optimal duration of risperidone or olanzapine adjunctive therapy to mood stabilizer following remission of a manic episode: a CANMAT randomized double-blind trial. Mol Psychiatry 2015. http://dx.doi.org/10.1038/mp.2015.158.

Drug-Induced Extrapyramidal Syndromes
Implications for Contemporary Practice

Stanley N. Caroff, MD[a],*, E. Cabrina Campbell, MD[b]

KEYWORDS

- Antipsychotic drugs • Schizophrenia • Tardive dyskinesia • Catatonia
- Neuroleptic malignant syndrome • Akathisia • Parkinsonism • Dystonia

KEY POINTS

- Awareness of acute drug-induced extrapyramidal syndromes (EPS) remains important for patient safety in clinical practice.
- Investigations of new treatments offer promise for managing patients with tardive dyskinesia.
- Advances in understanding the genetics and pathophysiology of EPS may illuminate the mechanisms of action of antipsychotic drugs and the biological bases of psychotic disorders.

INTRODUCTION

Although the origins of antipsychotic pharmacology began with the search for compounds to improve anesthesia, clinicians reported unusual "psychic indifference" as the defining effect of these drugs.[1] Nevertheless, early antipsychotics were thought to be useful primarily for sedation rather than specific antipsychotic effects, whereas drug-induced extrapyramidal syndromes (EPS) were considered necessary indicators that therapeutic doses had been achieved. Thus, the neurologic properties received pride of place in the original designation, "neuroleptics."

However, it soon became apparent that EPS can be mistaken for or worsen psychotic symptoms, are sometimes irreversible or lethal, necessitate additional burdensome adverse effects from antiparkinsonian agents, can be disfiguring and

Disclosure: Dr S.N. Caroff received a research grant from Sunovion Pharmaceuticals Inc and served as a consultant for Auspex Pharmaceuticals Inc.

[a] Department of Psychiatry, Perelman School of Medicine, University of Pennsylvania, 300 Blockley Hall, Philadelphia, PA 19104, USA; [b] Department of Psychiatry, Perelman School of Medicine, University of Pennsylvania, Corporal Michael J. Crescenz Veterans Affairs Medical Center-116A, University & Woodland Avenues, Philadelphia, PA 19104, USA
* Corresponding author. Department of Psychiatry, Perelman School of Medicine, University of Pennsylvania, 300 Blockley Hall, Philadelphia, PA, 19104.
E-mail address: caroffs@mail.med.upenn.edu

Abbreviations	
ECT	Electroconvulsive therapy
EPS	Extrapyramidal syndromes
FGA	First-generation antipsychotic
NMS	Neuroleptic malignant syndrome
SGA	Second-generation antipsychotic
TD	Tardive dyskinesia
VMAT2	Vesicular monoamine transporter type 2

stigmatizing, and may influence compliance, relapse, and rehospitalization.[2–4] As a result, EPS dominated concerns about tolerability of antipsychotics and drove new drug development.

In 1988, Kane and colleagues[5] reported that clozapine had broader efficacy in schizophrenia with negligible EPS, stimulating the search for new antipsychotics. Industry-sponsored trials heralded subsequent "second-generation antipsychotics" (SGAs) as superior to "first-generation antipsychotics" (FGAs) in causing fewer EPS.[6–13] Cumulative evidence, including the general consensus of clinicians, confirmed reduced liability for EPS with SGAs, contributing to their market dominance and the concept of "atypicality" in their mechanism of action.[14–21]

However, subsequent postmarketing studies challenged the advantages of SGAs in reducing EPS. The discrepancy between effectiveness and marketing trials stems from the choice of comparator drugs and dosages. Although haloperidol was a reasonable choice as a comparator in industry-sponsored trials as the first-line antipsychotic drug at the time, subsequent studies suggested that the advantages of SGAs in reducing EPS were diminished when lower doses or lower potency FGAs are used, or if prophylactic antiparkinsonian drugs are administered.[19,22–30] This implies that haloperidol is not paradigmatic of all FGAs; therefore, the dichotomy between first- and second generation drugs and the concept of SGA "atypicality" based on EPS liability was overstated. Antipsychotic drugs should be considered a single drug class with a spectrum of risk for EPS depending on dopamine D2 receptor binding affinity combined with affinity for other receptors.

Even though there is some reduction in risk of EPS with the SGAs, it remains important for clinicians to be familiar with EPS for several reasons. First, because dopamine D2 receptor blockade is preserved in all currently marketed antipsychotics and is necessary for antipsychotic efficacy, EPS remains a potential liability for all drugs in this class. Second, FGAs are still used in psychiatry, in medical settings, and in developing nations. Third, EPS must be balanced with risk for other significant adverse effects, for example, the metabolic syndrome. Fourth, the higher costs of newer drugs may be a consideration. Fifth, although the proportion of patients who develop EPS may be reduced, aggressive marketing and off-label prescribing contribute to an ever-widening population at risk. This development is especially concerning related to high-risk groups such as children, the elderly, and medically compromised patients. Familiarity with tardive dyskinesia (TD) is important because new drug treatments are likely to become available. In the future, genetic testing may uncover genetic susceptibilities to drug-induced EPS. Finally, research into EPS may provide insights into the mechanism of action of antipsychotic drugs. We, therefore, provide an updated review of the literature on diagnosis and management of the classic EPS syndromes including emerging evidence on treatment of TD.[1,30–32]

DYSTONIA
Clinical Features

Drug-induced dystonia is an acute movement disorder that can be painful and distressing, and can erode patient trust and medication adherence.[1,33,34] It is characterized by briefly sustained or intermittent spasms or contractions of antagonistic muscle groups resulting in twisting, sustained, and repetitive movements or postures. Drug-induced dystonia is usually focal and can affect any muscle group, but most commonly involves the head, neck, jaw, eyes, and mouth, resulting in spasmodic torticollis, retrocollis or anterocollis, trismus and dental trauma, forced jaw opening or dislocation, grimacing, blepharospasm, distortion of the lips, and tongue biting, protrusion, or twisting.[31,35,36] It is not clearly established whether it is action or sensory stimulus dependent. Subjective symptoms, including anxiety, muscle pain, cramps or tightness of the jaw, and tongue swelling with difficulty speaking or chewing, may precede dystonia or occur alone. Dystonia may also present as an oculogyric crisis or with other forced eye movements, or with dysarthria, dysphagia, or potentially lethal respiratory stridor if pharyngeal or laryngeal musculature is affected. Less frequently, dystonia may affect axial, truncal, or limb movements, occasionally leading to camptocormia (anterior flexion of the trunk), pleurothotonus or "Pisa syndrome" (lateral tilting of the trunk) or opisthotonus (arched extension of the trunk or spine).

Differential Diagnosis

The differential diagnosis of dystonia includes primary genetic disorders (eg, primary torsion dystonias) and secondary forms including neurodegenerative disorders (eg, Parkinson's disease), structural abnormalities of the brain (eg, after a stroke), and metabolic and toxic etiologies (eg, carbon monoxide poisoning).[34,36–38] Drug-induced dystonia is distinguished by associated drug treatment, negative family history, a focal and nonprogressive course, and absence of associated neurologic signs. Dystonia still may be diagnosed erroneously as conversion disorder if clinicians are unaware that dystonia can also fluctuate depending on whether the individual is stressed and anxious or is relaxed. On the other hand, some individuals may feign symptoms to avoid taking antipsychotic drugs or to abuse anticholinergic drugs.[35]

Course and Outcome

Dystonia is usually observed within a few hours of a single dose, especially after parenteral administration, but may appear after a delay of several hours to a few days.[31] In 95% of cases, dystonia appears within the first 5 days of treatment.[31,35] Although most often associated with drug initiation, dystonia may also occur when the dose is increased, a second antipsychotic is added, for the few days each time after long-acting injectable antipsychotics are administered, if another drug is added that inhibits antipsychotic metabolism, or after the discontinuation of antiparkinsonian agents. Dystonic reactions last a few seconds or several hours and may be sustained, fluctuating, or episodic.[1] After drug discontinuation, dystonia usually resolves within 24 to 48 hours.[36] Dystonia also occurs in a tardive form, which first appears or worsens when antipsychotics are discontinued. Dystonia occurs in 2% to 5% of patients receiving FGAs.[31,35,36] However, in young men receiving high-potency antipsychotics parenterally, the frequency approaches 90% in some studies.[31]

Risk Factors

Patient risk factors for dystonia include younger age, male gender, black race, previous dystonic reactions, family history of dystonia, cocaine use, mood disorders, hypocalcemia, hypoparathyroidism, hyperthyroidism, and dehydration.[35,36,39] Children and young adults are highly vulnerable and more likely to develop generalized dystonia, similar to the pattern in primary dystonias, whereas drug-induced dystonia is less common after 45 years of age.[35] Although knowledge of the genetics of primary idiopathic dystonias has progressed rapidly in recent years,[34,38,40] it remains unclear whether drug-induced dystonias are more likely to occur in people with the same genetic mutations that are found in families affected with primary dystonias.

Drug dosage, potency, and the rate of titration correlate with risk of dystonia.[35,36,41] Moderate to high doses of antipsychotics are associated with dystonia, whereas low or very high doses are involved less often.[1,39] Antipsychotics with weak dopamine antagonism and prominent anticholinergic (specifically, antimuscarinic) effects diminish the risk of dystonia, whereas the newer SGAs seem to have reduced liability as well.[14,15] Although haloperidol had up to a 4 times greater risk of causing dystonia than SGAs in industry-sponsored trials,[6,8,42] when the less potent FGA, perphenazine, was compared with SGAs in the Clinical Antipsychotic Trials of Intervention Effectiveness (CATIE) project, the rate of dystonia was only 0.4% overall, with no difference between treatment groups.[30] The CATIE data suggest that, in older patients with chronic schizophrenia, the use of a less potent FGA at modest doses presents no greater risk for dystonia than SGAs.

The advantages of SGAs over FGAs in reducing dystonia are also mitigated if an anticholingeric drug is given prophylactically along with the FGA.[33] However, using prophylactic anticholinergics can be problematic owing to adverse anticholinergic effects, which are especially hazardous in the elderly. But in young or other high-risk patients receiving parenteral, high-potency antipsychotics, or in paranoid or other patients ambivalent about treatment, the benefits of preventing dystonia with anticholinergics far outweigh potential risks.[43]

Treatment

Dystonia is responsive within 10 to 20 minutes to anticholinergic or antihistaminic agents administered parenterally. Benzodiazepines have been effective in some cases. If response is not achieved, a search for underlying disorders should be conducted or tardive dystonia considered.[44] After dystonia is suppressed, oral anticholinergics are continued for 24 to 48 hours if the antipsychotic is discontinued, or for at least several days if antipsychotic treatment is continued with gradual tapering to prevent recurrence. However, some patients may need continued prophylaxis, including those with a prior or recent history of dystonia or a history of particularly severe dystonic reactions, and those at higher risk such as young and male patients.

Pathophysiology

The exact pathophysiology of drug-induced dystonia is unresolved.[1,31,34,45] It remains unclear whether excessive dopaminergic activity from a compensatory increase in turnover after drug-induced receptor blockade causes dystonia as antipsychotic drug levels diminish (the "miss–match" hypothesis; ie, more dopamine being released presynaptically at the same time that postsynaptic dopamine receptor blockade declines), or whether dystonia results from dopamine antagonism per se, or from imbalances in relation to other neurotransmitters.[31] Recent clarification of the genetics of primary dystonia may shed light on mechanisms of drug-induced forms.[34,36,38,40]

PARKINSONISM
Clinical Features

Drug-induced parkinsonism is a subacute syndrome that mimics Parkinson's disease. Although less acute than dystonia, it is more common, more difficult to treat, and may cause significant disability, especially in the elderly. Patients may initially complain of fatigue, weakness, cognitive slowing, or depression.[1] Bradykinesia is prominent and accompanied by masked facies (hypomimia), reduced blink rate, positive glabellar tap (Myerson's sign), reduced arm swing, slowed initiation of activities, and dysphonic speech.[31] Bilateral and usually symmetrical rigidity of the neck, trunk, and extremities, which can be either "cog-wheel" or "lead-pipe" in tone, is a core finding. Resting, postural, or action tremors are also observed symmetrically and generalized, occasionally affecting the perioral muscles ("rabbit syndrome"). Patients may experience autonomic dysfunction, sialorrhea associated with dysphagia, postural changes (truncal hyperextension; ie, standing stiffly upright with a backward lean or "poker spine"), and gait disturbances (shuffling, festinating [ie, compulsive, small steps forward as if running], freezing [ie, hesitating to move], and anteropulsion or retropulsion [ie, difficulty stopping forward or backward motion]).[1]

Differential Diagnosis

It is important to differentiate drug-induced parkinsonism from negative symptoms of schizophrenia and psychomotor retardation associated with depression. It can be difficult to distinguish drug-induced from idiopathic parkinsonism. Parkinson's disease is more likely to be asymmetric, with an invariably progressive course, and is characterized by greater prominence of rigidity, tremor, and gait disturbance. Evidence of idiopathic disease may precede treatment and would not resolve even after antipsychotic drugs are discontinued. In contrast with patients with drug-induced forms, patients with Parkinson's disease show nigrostriatal degeneration on dopamine transporter scans and sympathetic dysregulation on iodine-123-metaiodobenzylguanidine cardiac scintigraphy.[46] Interestingly, olfactory deficits (hyposmia) have been reported in drug-induced parkinsonism and, therefore, may not be useful in differentiation from idiopathic parkinsonism, but may predict risk for prolonged symptoms after drug discontinuation owing to underlying Parkinson's disease.[47,48] The differential diagnosis also includes other causes of parkinsonism, including vascular parkinsonism, which also tends to be asymmetric.

Course and Outcome

Although dopamine receptor blockade occurs within hours after drug administration, the onset of parkinsonism may be delayed from days to weeks, with 50% to 75% of cases occurring within 1 month and 90% within 3 months.[31] Parkinsonism may also occur after doses are increased, a second antipsychotic is added, anticholinergic drugs are discontinued, or another drug is added that reduces dopamine activity or increases plasma levels of the antipsychotic. In most cases, symptoms are reversible in days or weeks, but occasionally, especially in the elderly, or if long-acting injectable antipsychotics are used, symptoms may last for months. In about 15% of cases, parkinsonism may persist after antipsychotic drug discontinuation, raising the possibility of underlying Parkinson's disease.[46,49]

Risk Factors

The incidence of drug-induced parkinsonism is variable depending on risk of the population studied, duration of follow-up, sensitivity of diagnosis, and potency of the drugs used, but has been estimated to occur in a range of 15% to 40% of patients treated with FGAs.[1,31] It is the second most common cause of parkinsonism after Parkinson's disease. The risk of drug-induced parkinsonism has been associated with advancing age, female gender, and abnormalities of brain structure including dementia, human immunodeficiency virus infection, and preexisting extrapyramidal disease or family history of Parkinson's disease.[31,46,50] Research on the genetics of susceptibility to drug-induced parkinsonism is limited, but offers the promise of identifying patients at risk, including those with underlying disease likely to be unmasked by drug treatment.[1,40,51]

Although parkinsonism has correlated with increased dosages and potency, and reduced anticholinergic properties of antipsychotics,[52] dose–response relationships have not always been clear in view of differences in individual susceptibility. Although haloperidol was associated with 2 to 4 times the risk of parkinsonism compared with SGAs (22%-38% vs 4%-14%) in industry trials,[6,8,14,15,42,53,54] there were no significant differences in the CATIE trial when perphenazine was compared with SGAs in the proportion of patients exhibiting parkinsonism, again suggesting that a less potent FGA at modest doses may present a similar risk compared with SGAs.[28–30]

Furthermore, judging by the severe motor worsening experienced by patients with Parkinson's disease after receiving antipsychotics, even SGAs may cause significant parkinsonism in susceptible individuals, with the exception of clozapine and quetiapine.[14,15] Patients with Lewy body dementia may experience a potentially lethal "neuroleptic sensitivity syndrome," which is characterized by worsening parkinsonism, confusion, sedation, and postural instability, when exposed to either FGAs or SGAs.[55]

Treatment

Prophylaxis of parkinsonism with anticholinergic drugs is less compelling than for dystonia and introduces significant risk of anticholinergic toxicity. Given the delayed onset of drug-induced parkinsonism, close monitoring for parkinsonian symptoms with prompt consideration of lowering dosages or switching to lower risk antipsychotics takes precedence, albeit with attendant risk of psychotic relapse. If a given antipsychotic is effective and cannot be changed, and if parkinsonism persists, treatment may include anticholinergic drugs or amantadine. However, there is surprisingly limited controlled evidence for the use of these agents.[44] Specific dopaminergic therapy is ineffective, owing to ongoing drug-induced blockade of dopamine receptors, and raises the risk of worsening psychotic symptoms. Once patients have been maintained on adjunctive antiparkinsonian therapy for 3 to 6 months, cautious tapering may be attempted.[31] However, several studies have shown that 62% to 96% of patients may still experience worsening parkinsonism after antiparkinsonian drug discontinuation.[56]

Pathophysiology

The mechanisms underlying drug-induced parkinsonism parallel Parkinson's disease itself.[1] Antipsychotics induce a functional dopamine deficiency in the corpus striatum by blocking dopamine receptors. Their liability for inducing parkinsonism, therefore, is the product of dopamine receptor binding affinity balanced by affinity for blocking muscarinic receptors.[52]

AKATHISIA
Clinical Features

Akathisia is another common drug-induced EPS.[1,31,50,57–60] However, akathisia is distinctive: it is defined as much by subjective as well as by objective features, it more often affects the lower extremities, it remains a frequent problem even with SGAs,[57] and it is more resistant to treatment. Subjectively, patients complain of inner tension, restlessness, anxiety, an urge to move, an inability to sit still, and drawing sensations in the legs. Motor features are complex, semipurposeful, and repetitive, including foot shuffling or tapping, shifting of weight, rocking, pacing incessantly, and even running. Although the severity of these sensations varies with stress and arousal, they can become intolerable and have been associated with violence and suicide.[57,59]

Differential Diagnosis

Acute drug-induced akathisia must be distinguished from tardive akathisia, neurodegenerative conditions, and drug-related states. Akathisia resembles restless legs syndrome, but the latter occurs during relaxation, rest, or sleep, mostly in the evening or night. Misdiagnosis of restless legs syndrome instead of drug-induced akathisia may lead to prescription of dopamine agonists, which could worsen psychosis in turn, leading to increased antipsychotic use, and further compounding akathisia.[58] Finally, distinguishing akathisia from agitation and anxiety can be challenging.

Course and Outcome

Akathisia may begin within several days after treatment but usually increases with duration of treatment, occurring in up to 50% of cases within 1 month and 90% of cases within 3 months.[31,60] Akathisia should resolve after drug discontinuation, but could temporarily worsen or persist in withdrawal or tardive forms.

Estimates of the incidence of akathisia vary from 21% to as high as 75% across studies of FGAs, with an estimated prevalence on average of at least 20% to 35% of patients depending on the susceptibility of the sample population, sensitivity of diagnosis, and the potency of drug treatment.[1,57,60]

Risk Factors

Risk factors for akathisia may include increasing age, female gender, negative symptoms, cognitive dysfunction, iron deficiency, prior akathisia, concomitant parkinsonism, and mood disorders.[1,58,59] There has been even less work on genetic susceptibility to akathisia compared with other EPS, but several genetic loci described in relation to restless legs syndrome may reveal common mechanisms.[1,40,61,62]

In most but not all clinical trials, SGAs have resulted in a significantly lower incidence of akathisia compared with FGAs.[57] Akathisia developed at a rate of about 2 to 7 times greater with haloperidol (15%-40%) compared with SGAs (0%-12%),[6,8,14,15,42,53,54] but when perphenazine rather than haloperidol was the comparator, there were no differences from SGAs in the incidence of akathisia.[28–30]

Treatment

There are no data on prophylaxis and, given its subacute onset, close observation for early signs is the best preventive measure. Once developed, akathisia should prompt reassessment of antipsychotic therapy, with a reduction in dosage, discontinuation, or switching to a less potent dopamine antagonist, all of which incur the risk of psychotic exacerbation or relapse. Evidence for the efficacy of treatments for akathisia derives mostly from small, short-term clinical trials without active comparative groups.[59,63] Lipophilic beta-adrenergic blockers have been effective in some studies, although limited by hypotension, bradycardia, and medical contraindications. Anticholinergics have been used traditionally, but evidence of their efficacy is limited; there were no randomized clinical trials that met inclusion criteria in a metaanalysis to support or refute their use in akathisia.[64] It has been suggested that anticholinergics may be more effective in the presence of concomitant parkinsonism, but this supposition is also untested.[1] Benzodiazepines have been useful owing to their anxiolytic and sedative properties. Amantadine may be effective in some cases. Recently, $5-HT_{2A}$ receptor antagonists have attracted interest, with mirtazapine showing equal efficacy and better tolerability in treating akathisia compared with propranolol.[59]

Pathophysiology

The pathophysiology of akathisia remains obscure, but dopamine antagonism underlying antipsychotic-induced akathisia, and treatment of restless legs syndrome with dopamine agonists, underscore the importance of dopamine-dependent mechanisms. Responses to beta-adrenergic and serotonergic blockers, suggest a role for other neurotransmitters as well.

CATATONIA

Clinical Features

Catatonia remains a continuing source of controversy as to its rightful place in psychiatric nosology.[65,66] However, it is essential for clinicians to be familiar with drug-induced catatonia and we include it here because, like drug-induced EPS syndromes, it is associated with antipsychotic drugs, it is characterized in part by abnormalities of posture and movement, and it mimics the well-known idiopathic form.

Catatonic symptoms that have been associated with antipsychotics include akinesia, rigidity, stupor, and mutism (akinetic mutism), and less often catalepsy and waxy flexibility.[67,68] More complex and qualitative catatonic behaviors typical of chronic psychotic disorders (stereotypies, echophenomena, verbigeration, automatic obedience) are rarely seen in drug-induced cases. In some patients, antipsychotics could transform preexisting catatonia into a more malignant form (malignant catatonia/neuroleptic malignant syndrome [NMS]).[69,70]

Differential Diagnosis

The differential diagnosis of catatonia includes a broad range of neurodegenerative, developmental, metabolic, toxic, infectious, and structural conditions affecting brain function.[71] Catatonia can occur in schizophrenia and mood disorders, or independently,[72] leading to the "catatonic dilemma,"[73] in which it may be difficult to distinguish primary catatonia from the effect of drug treatment itself. This dilemma may be resolved by discontinuing the antipsychotic medication, which leads to resolution of the catatonia in iatrogenic cases.

Course and Outcome

Drug-induced catatonia develops within hours to days and should resolve in a similar period of time after drug discontinuation. The onset of catatonia with antipsychotics has been reported to occur after discontinuation of concomitant benzodiazepines or antiparkinsonian agents. Only 5 cases of "catatonic neuroleptic syndrome" were reported among 86,439 patients receiving antipsychotics in a retrospective drug surveillance program.[74]

Risk Factors

Patient-related risk factors for drug-induced catatonia include past episodes and preexisting catatonic symptoms. Catatonia is observed mostly in association with high-potency drugs.[68] SGAs are not without risk; there are published case reports documenting both the occurrence and worsening of catatonia with SGAs, including precipitation of malignant catatonia or NMS.[14] However, SGAs have also been proposed as treatments for catatonia.[75,76]

Treatment

There are no data on whether prophylaxis with benzodiazepines or other agents may prevent catatonia. A more conservative approach would be to avoid using antipsychotics in catatonic patients, and to treat preexisting catatonia with benzodiazepines or electroconvulsive therapy (ECT). For patients at risk, clinicians should consider using other agents for the underlying psychiatric disorder, for example, lithium for mania. However, patients who require antipsychotic treatment merit careful monitoring. Treatment of drug-induced catatonia has not been studied, but must include reconsideration of the offending agent to prevent medical complications, including NMS. Specific treatment includes benzodiazepines, but some evidence suggests possible utility of amantadine or memantine.[68,77] Patients who fail to respond to these measures may require ECT.

Pathophysiology

The pathophysiology of drug-induced catatonia is unknown, but most likely involves drug effects on parallel dopamine pathways in basal ganglia-thalamocortical circuits subserving motor, arousal, volitional, and imitative behaviors.[78] Several investigators studied the genetic basis of idiopathic catatonia, which may correspond with drug sensitivity as well.[79–81]

NEUROLEPTIC MALIGNANT SYNDROME
Clinical Features

NMS represents an extremely rare but potentially lethal form of EPS combining features of advanced parkinsonism and catatonia.[4,82–84] Classic signs are hyperthermia, generalized rigidity with tremors, altered consciousness, and autonomic instability.[85] Rigidity is described as "lead pipe," tremors are often generalized, and other motor findings include dyskinesias, myoclonus, dysarthria, and dysphagia. In its extreme form, NMS presents as a hypermetabolic crisis with muscle enzyme elevations, myoglobinuria, leukocytosis, metabolic acidosis, hypoxia, elevated serum catecholamines, and low serum iron levels.

Differential Diagnosis

The differential diagnosis of NMS includes other disorders with increased temperatures and encephalopathy, such as malignant catatonia owing to psychosis,[70] central nervous system infections,[86,87] benign EPS, agitated delirium, heatstroke,[88] serotonin syndrome, stimulant intoxication, and withdrawal from dopamine agonists, sedatives, or alcohol. In the perioperative setting, NMS may be confused with malignant hyperthermia of anesthesia.[89] Although no laboratory test is diagnostic for NMS, a thorough assessment is necessary to exclude other serious medical conditions.

Course and Outcome

NMS may develop within hours but usually evolves over days; about two-thirds of cases occur during the first 1 to 2 weeks after drug initiation.[82] Once dopamine-blocking drugs are withheld, two-thirds of NMS cases resolve within 1 to 2 weeks, with an average duration of 7 to 10 days.[82] Patients may experience prolonged symptoms if injectable long-acting drugs are implicated. Occasional patients develop a residual catatonic/parkinsonian state after acute metabolic symptoms subside that can last for weeks to months unless ECT is administered.[90] If not recognized, NMS remains potentially fatal owing to renal failure, sudden cardiorespiratory arrest, disseminated intravascular coagulation, pulmonary emboli, or aspiration pneumonia.[91]

Risk Factors

The incidence of NMS is about 0.02% among patients treated with antipsychotic drugs.[74] Potential risk factors include dehydration, exhaustion, agitation, catatonia, previous episodes, and high doses of high-potency drugs given parenterally at a rapid rate.[82] The effect of concurrent use of multiple antipsychotics, lithium, and serotonin or serotonin–norepinephrine reuptake inhibitors on the risk of NMS has been suggested.[92] Most of these putative risk factors are commonly present and, therefore, of limited value in predicting NMS, which is a rare occurrence. The presence of such risk factors does not outweigh the value of antipsychotic drugs when they are indicated.

NMS has been associated with all antipsychotic drugs, but is more likely to occur with the use of high-potency agents. Haloperidol has accounted for about one-half of all reported cases. The SGAs have been implicated in case reports, but large-scale surveys suggest reduced risk compared with FGAs.[83,84] Atypical or milder forms have been reported in association with SGAs, but NMS has always varied in severity even with FGAs.

Treatment

The management of NMS consists of early diagnosis, discontinuing dopamine antagonists, and providing supportive medical care. In addition to these general measures, the use of benzodiazepines, dopamine agonists, dantrolene, and ECT have been advocated, but controlled trials comparing these agents may not be feasible because NMS is rare, often self-limited after drug discontinuation, and heterogeneous in presentation, course, and outcome.[83] We proposed that these agents be considered empirically in individual cases, and based on symptoms, severity, and duration of the episode.[83]

Pathophysiology

Several lines of evidence strongly implicate drug-induced dopamine receptor blockade as the primary triggering mechanism in the pathogenesis of NMS.[78] However, the involvement of other neurotransmitter systems and alternative autonomic or neuromuscular hypotheses have also been proposed.[93] Genetic findings have been reported in case reports, but without consistent results.

TARDIVE DYSKINESIA
Clinical Features

In contrast with acute EPS, TD is insidious in onset, arises after prolonged antipsychotic treatment, and is often masked by ongoing treatment. TD is irreversible in most cases, but usually mild, whereas acute EPS are transient but unmistakable and incapacitating.[1] Even so, TD can become socially disfiguring and compromise eating, speaking, breathing, or ambulation. Although the risk of TD may have decreased with SGAs, it is not absent, and it persists as a legacy of treatment with FGAs for thousands of patients.

TD presents as a polymorphous, involuntary movement disorder.[31,94,95] Unlike the reaction to acute EPS, subjective symptoms are often described as minimal or denied by patients with TD, at least in mild cases. In the CATIE trial of chronic schizophrenia, patients were 10 times more likely to discontinue treatment because of acute EPS compared with TD.[29,96] However, in more functional patients, or in those with severe dyskinesias, TD can be quite disturbing and emotionally intolerable. In its most common choreoathetoid form, the motor signs of TD are heterogeneous, involuntary, non-rhythmic, repetitive, purposeless, and hyperkinetic. In 60% to 80% of patients, TD primarily affects orofacial and lingual musculature ("buccolinguomasticatory syndrome") with chewing or bruxism of the jaw; protrusion, curling, twisting, or vermicular movements of the tongue; lip smacking, puckering, sucking and pursing, and retraction; grimacing or bridling of the mouth; bulging of the cheeks; or eye blinking and blepharospasm.[1,31] Choreoathetoid movements of the fingers, hands, and upper or lower extremities are common. Axial symptoms affecting the neck, shoulders, spine, or pelvis may be observed.

Tardive movements other than the classical choreoathetoid dyskinesias may develop as the predominant feature or in combinations with other movement types. These other movements, such as tardive dystonia, may represent subtypes of a tardive syndrome and may be associated with increased risk of progression, persistence, and severe disability. For example, tardive dystonia, estimated to occur in 3% to 5% of treated patients,[1,44,97] may be more generalized and disabling than TD, and may respond to anticholinergic agents. Akathisia, tics, and other movement disorders also occur as tardive variants.[98] Dyskinesias increase with emotional arousal, activation, or distraction, and diminish with relaxation, sleep, or volitional effort. As a result, symptoms of TD fluctuate over time, such that repeated measurements are necessary for reliable assessment of severity and persistence.

Differential Diagnosis

A neurologic evaluation is indicated for new-onset dyskinesias. Clues to primary neurologic causes include family history, sudden onset or progressive course, and associated medical or neurologic abnormalities. TD can be symmetric or unilateral. The differential diagnosis of TD includes neurodegenerative disorders, structural abnormalities of the brain, and metabolic and toxic etiologies. Persistent TD may be difficult to distinguish from acute EPS, transient withdrawal dyskinesias, or spontaneous dyskinesias associated with schizophrenia and aging.

Course and Outcome

The onset of TD occurs insidiously over 3 months or more of treatment and may begin with ticlike orofacial or lingual movements or increased eye blink frequency. TD is suppressed or masked by ongoing antipsychotic treatment, becoming apparent only when treatment is reduced, switched, or discontinued.

The natural course of TD has become increasingly clear. Early studies showed that withdrawal of antipsychotics may lead to an initial worsening of TD in 33% to 53% of patients, but 36% to 55% of patients eventually improve, which led to recommendations for drug reduction or withdrawal.[99] However, complete and permanent reversibility beyond the withdrawal period may be uncommon.[100,101] In a metaanalysis, Soares and McGrath[102] reported that 37.3% of patients assigned to placebo across studies showed some improvement in TD, but concluded that evidence was insufficient to support antipsychotic drug cessation or dose reduction in view of the risk for psychotic relapse.

Data on the prevalence of TD during continued treatment with antipsychotics have been inconclusive, with some studies showing an increase and others a decrease or no change at all.[96] Roughly 50% of patients have persistent TD symptoms, 10% to 30% have a reduction, and 10% to 30% show increased symptoms during continued treatment.[103] Long-term studies estimated that between 2% and 23% of patients show loss of observable TD symptoms during treatment with FGAs.[96] Similarly, studies of SGAs have generally shown reduction of TD ratings over time during the course of treatment, with some studies showing greater or lesser reductions and some showing no difference in comparison with FGAs.[96] Improved outcome of TD correlates in some studies with younger age, lower doses, reduced duration of drug treatment and of dyskinesia, and increased duration of follow-up.

The CATIE trial added important data on the course of TD during antipsychotic treatment; there was a significant decline in TD severity among patients with TD at baseline who were randomized to treatment with SGAs, but there were no significant differences between SGAs in the decline in ratings.[96] Of these patients who had TD at baseline, 55% continued to meet criteria for TD at 2 consecutive visits after baseline, 76% met criteria at some or all postbaseline visits, 24% did not meet criteria at any subsequent visit, and 32% showed at least a 50% decrease and 7% showed at least a 50% increase in AIMS scores compared with baseline ratings. Thus, most of the patients who already had TD before randomization showed either persistence or fluctuation in observable symptoms during the trial.

Risk Factors

The risk of TD has been extensively studied; several studies have shown a cumulative incidence of TD of about 4% to 5% annually, with a prevalence rate of 20% to 25%.[94] In studies of first episode patients, the incidence of TD was 6% to 12% in the first year even when low doses of antipsychotics were used.[104,105] The annual incidence of TD in patients over the age of 45 years was 15% to 30% after 1 year of treatment, with a prevalence rate of up to 50% to 60%.[106] Previous studies of TD risk have suggested an association with increasing age, female gender, psychiatric diagnosis, longer duration of antipsychotic treatment, greater cumulative drug doses, concomitant drug treatments, higher ratings of negative symptoms and thought disorder, greater cognitive impairments, presence of acute EPS, substance abuse, and diabetes.[107]

An increasing number of genes have been studied in TD based on theories of pathogenesis, including neurotransmitter metabolism and receptor dysfunction, enzymes protecting against oxidative stress, and pharmacokinetics.[1,40,108] In relation to proposed treatment of TD with tetrabenazine, a vesicular monoamine transporter type 2 (VMAT2) inhibitor, an association between ratings of TD and a single nucleotide polymorphism in the gene encoding VMAT2 was reported recently.[109] Although an association for this VMAT2 marker with TD was found among candidate genes studied in the CATIE trial,[110] no single marker or haplotype association attained statistical significance in this analysis. In a genome-wide association study of the same sample of CATIE patients, a single nucleotide polymorphism different from the VMAT2 marker was associated significantly with ratings of dyskinesias on the AIMS.[111] Further investigations are needed to test the validity of these genetic predispositions mediating TD.

Differences in liability for TD between FGAs and SGAs have been studied extensively. Compared with the incidence of TD with haloperidol, industry-sponsored trials of SGAs found a 6- to 12-fold reduction in risk for TD.[12,27,112–114] It remains questionable whether clozapine causes TD at all.[115] In contrast with industry studies using haloperidol, in the CATIE trial there were no differences in the incidence of TD among groups receiving perphenazine or SGAs.[28,29]

Treatment

Because there is no proven treatment for TD, it is important to minimize the risk by prevention and early detection (**Fig. 1**). Some preventive principles are to confirm the indication for antipsychotics, use conservative doses opting for lower potency agents, inform patients and caregivers of risk, assess on a regular basis for incipient signs,

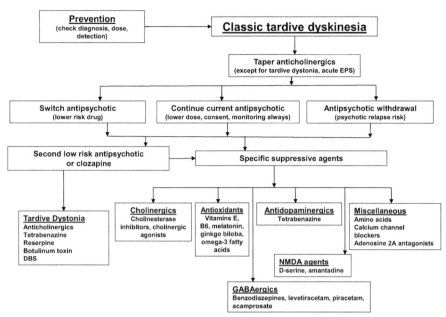

Fig. 1. Treatment algorithm for tardive dyskinesia. DBS, deep brain stimulation; EPS, extra-pyramidal syndromes; NMDA, *N*-methyl-D-aspartate. (*Adapted from* Caroff SN, Hurford I, Lybrand J, et al. Movement disorders induced by antipsychotic drugs: implications of the CATIE schizophrenia trial. Neurol Clin 2011;29:140; with permission.)

and consider differential diagnosis and reconsider drug treatment if symptoms emerge.

Once TD is detected, the first concern of management is to decide about antipsychotic treatment. Although drug withdrawal had been recommended in the past, about 33% to 53% of patients will experience worsening of dyskinesias initially, 36% to 55% may show improvement over time,[99] but few will show complete resolution of symptoms,[101] and patients with schizophrenia incur a significant risk of psychotic relapse. In patients without an underlying psychotic disorder, such as those who develop TD while taking dopamine antagonists like metoclopramide for nonpsychiatric reasons, drug continuation may be difficult to justify.

A second option in a patient who requires antipsychotic therapy and has good control of psychotic symptoms is to reduce the dose of antipsychotic gradually, inform patients of risks, document the decision, and monitor carefully. In most cases, TD is not progressive even with continued antipsychotic treatment, although symptoms may worsen in some cases.[96] Another alternative is to switch antipsychotics; more potent FGA antipsychotics suppress symptoms of TD in about 67% of patients, although limiting recovery and exacerbating acute EPS.[103] Switching to SGAs has also been associated with reduction of TD symptoms.[14,15] The CATIE trial provided direct evidence that randomization to an SGA resulted in a significant decline in mean ratings of TD severity.[96] Although most patients who had TD at baseline and were randomized to SGAs showed a persistent (34%) or fluctuating course (42%), 24% did not meet criteria on any visit at follow-up, and 32% showed a greater than 50% reduction in TD scores, whereas only 7% showed increased ratings.[96] Clozapine has been recommended for suppressing TD, especially the tardive dystonia variant.[116] Existing data are inconclusive as to whether recovery rather than simply suppression occurs during treatment with SGAs or FGAs.

If anticholinergic drugs have been prescribed, a decision also should be made about whether continuation is necessary or gradual tapering could be considered. Anticholinergic drugs probably worsen TD generally, such that improvement in TD severity ratings has been noted in up to 60% of patients withdrawn from these agents.[103] However, anticholinergic drugs may have been prescribed for concurrent acute EPS or for tardive dystonia, which are likely to worsen after anticholinergic withdrawal.

Pathophysiology

Apart from optimizing antipsychotic and anticholinergic therapy, there are a large number of specific agents under investigation for the treatment of TD based on competing theories of pathogenesis (see **Fig. 1**).[1,103,117–119] For example, antioxidants have been studied based on findings that drug-induced dopamine receptor blockade increases production of free radicals, which in turn may cause neuronal damage underlying TD.[119]

The hypothesis of dopamine supersensitivity may explain the suppressive effects of dopamine antagonists on TD, and has rekindled interest in tetrabenazine, which depletes presynaptic dopamine by inhibiting VMAT2, as a treatment for TD. Observational studies showing its suppressive effect in TD are being confirmed in controlled trials.[119–121] Based on evidence of antipsychotic drug-induced striatal glutaminergic hyperactivity underlying TD, and reported benefits in treating levodopa-induced dyskinesias, amantadine is also under study.[118,122]

Another hypothesis proposes that TD results from diminished cholinergic activity owing to damage of striatal cholinergic interneurons after the loss of dopamine-mediated inhibition.[123–125] Indirect support stems from the observation that anticholinergic agents probably worsen TD.[103] We inferred that cholinesterase inhibitors or cholinergic agonists may be effective in suppressing TD by directly enhancing postsynaptic cholinergic activity, compensating for the loss of presynaptic cholinergic neurons. Preliminary trials have explored the use of cholinesterase inhibitors with mixed results.[124,125] However, cholinesterase inhibitors nonspecifically increase cholinergic activity at multiple receptors, whereas more recent studies have shown beneficial effects of specific nicotine and muscarinic agonists on both levodopa-induced and antipsychotic-induced dyskinesias in animal models, suggesting that further investigations of specific nicotinic and muscarinic agonists in TD may be worthwhile.[126–128]

SUMMARY

New antipsychotics allow clinicians to tailor pharmacotherapy to the needs and vulnerabilities of individual patients. Antipsychotics should be conceptualized as a single drug class with a spectrum of risk for EPS depending on their receptor binding profile and individual patient susceptibility. Notwithstanding whether SGAs have reduced liability for EPS because of weaker dopamine receptor affinity or "atypical" mechanisms, their dominance in clinical practice has reduced significantly the frequency of EPS. However, knowledge of drug-induced EPS remains important for medicolegal and clinical reasons, and a better understanding of their pathophysiology and genetics may provide insights into the mechanism of action of antipsychotics and the biological basis of psychotic disorders. Continued study of TD is especially important and a moral imperative, given that treatments are being developed that offer new hope for thousands of patients left with dyskinesias as a legacy of antipsychotic treatment.

REFERENCES

1. Owens DGC. A guide to the extrapyramidal side-effects of antipsychotic drugs. 2nd edition. Cambridge (United Kingdom): Cambridge University Press; 2014.
2. Van Putten T. Why do schizophrenic patients refuse to take their drugs? Arch Gen Psychiatry 1975;31:67–72.
3. Rifkin A. Extrapyramidal side effects: a historical perspective. J Clin Psychiatry 1987;48(Suppl):3–6.
4. Caroff S. The neuroleptic malignant syndrome. J Clin Psychiatry 1980;41:79–83.
5. Kane J, Honigfeld G, Singer J, et al. Clozapine for the treatment-resistant schizophrenic. A double-blind comparison with chlorpromazine. Arch Gen Psychiatry 1988;45(9):789–96.
6. Arvanitis LA, Miller BG. Multiple fixed doses of "Seroquel" (quetiapine) in patients with acute exacerbation of schizophrenia: a comparison with haloperidol and placebo. The Seroquel Trial 13 Study Group. Biol Psychiatry 1997;42(4): 233–46.
7. Potkin SG, Saha AR, Kujawa MJ, et al. Aripiprazole, an antipsychotic with a novel mechanism of action, and risperidone vs placebo in patients with schizophrenia and schizoaffective disorder. Arch Gen Psychiatry 2003;60(7):681–90.
8. Tollefson GD, Beasley CM Jr, Tran PV, et al. Olanzapine versus haloperidol in the treatment of schizophrenia and schizoaffective and schizophreniform disorders: results of an international collaborative trial. Am J Psychiatry 1997;154(4): 457–65.
9. Marder SR, Meibach RC. Risperidone in the treatment of schizophrenia. Am J Psychiatry 1994;151(6):825–35.
10. Daniel DG, Zimbroff DL, Potkin SG, et al. Ziprasidone 80 mg/day and 160 mg/day in the acute exacerbation of schizophrenia and schizoaffective disorder: a 6-week placebo-controlled trial. Ziprasidone Study Group. Neuropsychopharmacology 1999;20(5):491–505.
11. Dossenbach M, Arango-Davila C, Silva Ibarra H, et al. Response and relapse in patients with schizophrenia treated with olanzapine, risperidone, quetiapine, or haloperidol: 12-month follow-up of the intercontinental schizophrenia outpatient health outcomes (IC-SOHO) study. J Clin Psychiatry 2005;66(8):1021–30.
12. Correll CU, Leucht S, Kane JM. Lower risk for tardive dyskinesia associated with second-generation antipsychotics: a systematic review of 1-year studies. Am J Psychiatry 2004;161(3):414–25.
13. Tenback DE, van Harten PN, Slooff CJ, et al. Effects of antipsychotic treatment on tardive dyskinesia: a 6-month evaluation of patients from the European schizophrenia outpatient health outcomes (SOHO) study. J Clin Psychiatry 2005;66(9):1130–3.
14. Caroff SN, Mann SC, Campbell EC, et al. Movement disorders associated with atypical antipsychotic drugs. J Clin Psychiatry 2002;63(Suppl 4):12–9.
15. Tarsy D, Baldessarini RJ, Tarazi FI. Effects of newer antipsychotics on extrapyramidal function. CNS Drugs 2002;16(1):23–45.
16. Kane JM, Woerner M, Lieberman J. Tardive dyskinesia: prevalence, incidence, and risk factors. J Clin Psychopharmacol 1988;8(4 Suppl):52S–6S.
17. Glazer WM. Expected incidence of tardive dyskinesia associated with atypical antipsychotics. J Clin Psychiatry 2000;61(Suppl 4):21–6.
18. Glazer WM. Extrapyramidal side effects, tardive dyskinesia, and the concept of atypicality. J Clin Psychiatry 2000;61(Suppl 3):16–21.

19. Leucht S, Pitschel-Walz G, Abraham D, et al. Efficacy and extrapyramidal side-effects of the new antipsychotics olanzapine, quetiapine, risperidone, and sertindole compared to conventional antipsychotics and placebo. A meta-analysis of randomized controlled trials. Schizophr Res 1999;35(1):51–68.
20. Meltzer HY. The mechanism of action of novel antipsychotic drugs. Schizophr Bull 1991;17(2):263–87.
21. Davis JM, Chen N, Glick ID. A meta-analysis of the efficacy of second-generation antipsychotics. Arch Gen Psychiatry 2003;60(6):553–64.
22. Geddes J, Freemantle N, Harrison P, et al. Atypical antipsychotics in the treatment of schizophrenia: systematic overview and meta-regression analysis. BMJ 2000;321(7273):1371–6.
23. Leucht S, Wahlbeck K, Hamann J, et al. New generation antipsychotics versus low-potency conventional antipsychotics: a systematic review and meta-analysis. Lancet 2003;361(9369):1581–9.
24. Rosenheck R, Perlick D, Bingham S, et al. Effectiveness and cost of olanzapine and haloperidol in the treatment of schizophrenia: a randomized controlled trial. JAMA 2003;290(20):2693–702.
25. Hugenholtz GW, Heerdink ER, Stolker JJ, et al. Haloperidol dose when used as active comparator in randomized controlled trials with atypical antipsychotics in schizophrenia: comparison with officially recommended doses. J Clin Psychiatry 2006;67(6):897–903.
26. Jones PB, Barnes TR, Davies L, et al. Randomized controlled trial of the effect on quality of life of second- vs first-generation antipsychotic drugs in schizophrenia: cost utility of the latest antipsychotic drugs in schizophrenia study (CUtLASS 1). Arch Gen Psychiatry 2006;63(10):1079–87.
27. Correll CU, Schenk EM. Tardive dyskinesia and new antipsychotics. Curr Opin Psychiatry 2008;21(2):151–6.
28. Lieberman JA, Stroup TS, McEvoy JP, et al. Effectiveness of antipsychotic drugs in patients with chronic schizophrenia. N Engl J Med 2005;353(12):1209–23.
29. Miller DD, Caroff SN, Davis SM, et al. Extrapyramidal side-effects of antipsychotics in a randomised trial. Br J Psychiatry 2008;193(4):279–88.
30. Caroff SN, Miller DD, Rosenheck RA. Extrapyramidal side effects. In: Stroup TS, Lieberman JA, editors. The Clinical Antipsychotic Trials of Intervention Effectiveness (CATIE) schizophrenia trial: how does it inform practice, policy, and research? Cambridge (United Kingdom): Cambridge University Press; 2010. p. 156–72.
31. Tarsy D. Neuroleptic-induced extrapyramidal reactions: classification, description, and diagnosis. Clin Neuropharmacol 1983;6(Suppl 1):S9–26.
32. Caroff SN, Hurford I, Lybrand J, et al. Movement disorders induced by antipsychotic drugs: implications of the CATIE schizophrenia trial. Neurol Clin 2011; 29(1):127–48.
33. Satterthwaite TD, Wolf DH, Rosenheck RA, et al. A meta-analysis of the risk of acute extrapyramidal symptoms with intramuscular antipsychotics for the treatment of agitation. J Clin Psychiatry 2008;69(12):1869–79.
34. Tarsy D, Simon DK. Dystonia. N Engl J Med 2006;355(8):818–29.
35. van Harten PN, Hoek HW, Kahn RS. Acute dystonia induced by drug treatment. BMJ 1999;319(7210):623–6.
36. Rupniak NM, Jenner P, Marsden CD. Acute dystonia induced by neuroleptic drugs. Psychopharmacology (Berl) 1986;88(4):403–19.
37. Marsden CD, Quinn NP. The dystonias. BMJ 1990;300(6718):139–44.

38. Nemeth AH. The genetics of primary dystonias and related disorders. Brain 2002;125(Pt 4):695–721.
39. Keepers GA, Casey DE. Prediction of neuroleptic-induced dystonia. J Clin Psychopharmacol 1987;7(5):342–5.
40. Crisafulli C, Drago A, Sidoti A, et al. A genetic dissection of antipsychotic induced movement disorders. Curr Med Chem 2013;20(3):312–30.
41. Keepers GA, Clappison VJ, Casey DE. Initial anticholinergic prophylaxis for neuroleptic-induced extrapyramidal syndromes. Arch Gen Psychiatry 1983; 40(10):1113–7.
42. Simpson GM, Lindenmayer JP. Extrapyramidal symptoms in patients treated with risperidone. J Clin Psychopharmacol 1997;17(3):194–201.
43. Arana GW, Goff DC, Baldessarini RJ, et al. Efficacy of anticholinergic prophylaxis for neuroleptic-induced acute dystonia. Am J Psychiatry 1988;145(8): 993–6.
44. Dayalu P, Chou KL. Antipsychotic-induced extrapyramidal symptoms and their management. Expert Opin Pharmacother 2008;9(9):1451–62.
45. Berardelli A, Rothwell JC, Hallett M, et al. The pathophysiology of primary dystonia. Brain 1998;121(Pt 7):1195–212.
46. Thanvi B, Treadwell S. Drug induced parkinsonism: a common cause of parkinsonism in older people. Postgrad Med J 2009;85(1004):322–6.
47. Bovi T, Antonini A, Ottaviani S, et al. The status of olfactory function and the striatal dopaminergic system in drug-induced parkinsonism. J Neurol 2010;257(11): 1882–9.
48. Morley JF, Duda JE. Use of hyposmia and other non-motor symptoms to distinguish between drug-induced parkinsonism and Parkinson's disease. J Parkinsons Dis 2014;4(2):169–73.
49. Morley JF, Pawlowski SM, Kesari A, et al. Motor and non-motor features of Parkinson's disease that predict persistent drug-induced Parkinsonism. Parkinsonism Relat Disord 2014;20(7):738–42.
50. Gelenberg AJ. General principles of treatment of extrapyramidal syndromes. Clin Neuropharmacol 1983;6(Suppl 1):S52–6.
51. Bras JM, Singleton A. Genetic susceptibility in Parkinson's disease. Biochim Biophys Acta 2009;1792(7):597–603.
52. Snyder S, Greenberg D, Yamamura HI. Antischizophrenic drugs and brain cholinergic receptors. Affinity for muscarinic sites predicts extrapyramidal effects. Arch Gen Psychiatry 1974;31(1):58–61.
53. Hirsch SR, Kissling W, Bauml J, et al. A 28-week comparison of ziprasidone and haloperidol in outpatients with stable schizophrenia. J Clin Psychiatry 2002; 63(6):516–23.
54. Barnes TR, McPhillips MA. Critical analysis and comparison of the side-effect and safety profiles of the new antipsychotics. Br J Psychiatry Suppl 1999;38: 34–43.
55. McKeith IG, Dickson DW, Lowe J, et al. Diagnosis and management of dementia with Lewy bodies: third report of the DLB consortium. Neurology 2005;65(12): 1863–72.
56. Gelenberg AJ. Treating extrapyramidal reactions: some current issues. J Clin Psychiatry 1987;48(Suppl):24–7.
57. Kane JM, Fleischhacker WW, Hansen L, et al. Akathisia: an updated review focusing on second-generation antipsychotics. J Clin Psychiatry 2009;70(5): 627–43.

58. Bratti IM, Kane JM, Marder SR. Chronic restlessness with antipsychotics. Am J Psychiatry 2007;164(11):1648–54.
59. Poyurovsky M. Acute antipsychotic-induced akathisia revisited. Br J Psychiatry 2010;196(2):89–91.
60. Sachdev P, Kruk J. Clinical characteristics and predisposing factors in acute drug-induced akathisia. Arch Gen Psychiatry 1994;51(12):963–74.
61. Eichhammer P, Albus M, Borrmann-Hassenbach M, et al. Association of dopamine D3-receptor gene variants with neuroleptic induced akathisia in schizophrenic patients: a generalization of Steen's study on DRD3 and tardive dyskinesia. Am J Med Genet 2000;96(2):187–91.
62. Pichler I, Hicks AA, Pramstaller PP. Restless legs syndrome: an update on genetics and future perspectives. Clin Genet 2008;73(4):297–305.
63. Miller CH, Fleischhacker WW. Managing antipsychotic-induced acute and chronic akathisia. Drug Saf 2000;22(1):73–81.
64. Rathbone J, Soares-Weiser K. Anticholinergics for neuroleptic-induced acute akathisia. Cochrane Database Syst Rev 2006;(4):CD003727.
65. Ungvari GS, Caroff SN, Gerevich J. The catatonia conundrum: evidence of psychomotor phenomena as a symptom dimension in psychotic disorders. Schizophr Bull 2010;36(2):231–8.
66. Ungvari GS. Catatonia in DSM 5: controversies regarding its psychopathology, clinical presentation and treatment response. Neuropsychopharmacol Hung 2014;16(4):189–94.
67. Lopez-Canino A, Francis A. Drug-induced catatonia. In: Caroff SN, Mann SC, Francis A, et al, editors. Catatonia: from psychopathology to neurobiology. Washington, DC: American Psychiatric Press, Inc.; 2004. p. 129–39.
68. Gelenberg AJ, Mandel MR. Catatonic reactions to high-potency neuroleptic drugs. Arch Gen Psychiatry 1977;34(8):947–50.
69. White DA, Robins AH. An analysis of 17 catatonic patients diagnosed with neuroleptic malignant syndrome. CNS Spectr 2000;5(7):58–65.
70. Mann SC, Caroff SN, Bleier HR, et al. Lethal catatonia. Am J Psychiatry 1986; 143(11):1374–81.
71. Gelenberg AJ. The catatonic syndrome. Lancet 1976;1(7973):1339–41.
72. Caroff SN, Hurford I, Bleier HR, et al. Recurrent idiopathic catatonia: implications beyond the diagnostic and statistical manual of mental disorders 5th edition. Clin Psychopharmacol Neurosci 2015;13(2):218–21.
73. Brenner I, Rheuban WJ. The catatonic dilemma. Am J Psychiatry 1978;135(10): 1242–3.
74. Stubner S, Rustenbeck E, Grohmann R, et al. Severe and uncommon involuntary movement disorders due to psychotropic drugs. Pharmacopsychiatry 2004; 37(Suppl 1):S54–64.
75. Van Den Eede F, Van Hecke J, Van Dalfsen A, et al. The use of atypical antipsychotics in the treatment of catatonia. Eur Psychiatry 2005;20(5–6):422–9.
76. Peralta V, Campos MS, de Jalon EG, et al. DSM-IV catatonia signs and criteria in first-episode, drug-naive, psychotic patients: psychometric validity and response to antipsychotic medication. Schizophr Res 2010;118(1–3):168–75.
77. Carroll BT, Goforth HW, Thomas C, et al. Review of adjunctive glutamate antagonist therapy in the treatment of catatonic syndromes. J Neuropsychiatry Clin Neurosci 2007;19(4):406–12.
78. Mann SC, Caroff SN, Fricchione G, et al. Central dopamine hypoactivity and the pathogenesis of neuroleptic malignant syndrome. Psychiatr Ann 2000;30: 363–74.

79. Stober G. Genetics. In: Caroff SN, Mann SC, Francis A, et al, editors. Catatonia: from psychopathology to neurobiology. Washington, DC: American Psychiatric Press, Inc; 2004. p. 173–87.

80. Ehrenreich H, Nave KA. Phenotype-based genetic association studies (PGAS)-towards understanding the contribution of common genetic variants to schizophrenia subphenotypes. Genes (Basel) 2014;5(1):97–105.

81. Kanes SJ. Animal models. In: Caroff SN, Mann SC, Francis A, et al, editors. Catatonia: from psychopathology to neurobiology. Washington, DC: American Psychiatric Press, Inc.; 2004. p. 189–200.

82. Caroff SN, Mann SC. Neuroleptic malignant syndrome. Med Clin North Am 1993;77(1):185–202.

83. Strawn JR, Keck PE Jr, Caroff SN. Neuroleptic malignant syndrome. Am J Psychiatry 2007;164(6):870–6.

84. Caroff SN, Mann SC, Campbell EC, et al. Severe drug reactions. In: Ferrando SJ, Levenson JL, Owen JA, editors. Clinical manual of psychopharmacology in the medically III. Washington, DC: American Psychiatric Press, Inc.; 2010. p. 39–77.

85. Gurrera RJ, Caroff SN, Cohen A, et al. An international consensus study of neuroleptic malignant syndrome diagnostic criteria using the Delphi method. J Clin Psychiatry 2011;72(9):1222–8.

86. Caroff SN, Mann SC, McCarthy M, et al. Acute infectious encephalitis complicated by neuroleptic malignant syndrome. J Clin Psychopharmacol 1998; 18(4):349–51.

87. Caroff SN, Campbell EC. Risk of neuroleptic malignant syndrome in patients with NMDAR encephalitis. Neurol Sci 2015;36(3):479–80.

88. Mann SC, Boger WP. Psychotropic drugs, summer heat and humidity, and hyperpyrexia: a danger restated. Am J Psychiatry 1978;135(9):1097–100.

89. Caroff SN, Rosenberg H, Mann SC, et al. Neuroleptic malignant syndrome in the perioperative setting. Am J Anesthesiol 2001;28:387–93.

90. Caroff SN, Mann SC, Keck PE Jr, et al. Residual catatonic state following neuroleptic malignant syndrome. J Clin Psychopharmacol 2000;20(2):257–9.

91. Modi S, Dharaiya D, Schultz L, et al. Neuroleptic malignant syndrome: complications, outcomes, and mortality. Neurocrit Care 2016;24(1):97–103.

92. Stevens DL. Association between selective serotonin-reuptake inhibitors, second-generation antipsychotics, and neuroleptic malignant syndrome. Ann Pharmacother 2008;42(9):1290–7.

93. Gurrera RJ. Sympathoadrenal hyperactivity and the etiology of neuroleptic malignant syndrome. Am J Psychiatry 1999;156(2):169–80.

94. Kane JM. Tardive dyskinesia: epidemiological and clinical presentation. In: Bloom FE, Kupfer DJ, editors. Psychopharmacology: the fourth generation of progress. New York: Raven Press; 1995. p. 1485–95.

95. Casey DE. Neuroleptic drug-induced extrapyramidal syndromes and tardive dyskinesia. Schizophr Res 1991;4(2):109–20.

96. Caroff SN, Davis VG, Miller DD, et al. Treatment outcomes of patients with tardive dyskinesia and chronic schizophrenia. J Clin Psychiatry 2011;72(3): 295–303.

97. Adityanjee, Aderibigbe YA, Jampala VC, et al. The current status of tardive dystonia. Biol Psychiatry 1999;45(6):715–30.

98. Burke RE, Kang UJ, Jankovic J, et al. Tardive akathisia: an analysis of clinical features and response to open therapeutic trials. Mov Disord 1989;4(2):157–75.

99. Casey DE, Gerlach J. Tardive dyskinesia: what is the long-term outcome?. In: Casey DE, Gardos G, editors. Tardive dyskinesia and neuroleptics: from dogma to reason. Washington, DC: American Psychiatric Press, Inc.; 1986. p. 76–97.

100. Glazer WM, Moore DC, Schooler NR, et al. Tardive dyskinesia. A discontinuation study. Arch Gen Psychiatry 1984;41(6):623–7.

101. Glazer WM, Morgenstern H, Schooler N, et al. Predictors of improvement in tardive dyskinesia following discontinuation of neuroleptic medication. Br J Psychiatry 1990;157:585–92.

102. Soares KV, McGrath JJ. The treatment of tardive dyskinesia–a systematic review and meta-analysis. Schizophr Res 1999;39(1):1–16 [discussion: 17–8].

103. Egan MF, Apud J, Wyatt RJ. Treatment of tardive dyskinesia. Schizophr Bull 1997;23(4):583–609.

104. Chakos MH, Alvir JM, Woerner MG, et al. Incidence and correlates of tardive dyskinesia in first episode of schizophrenia. Arch Gen Psychiatry 1996;53(4):313–9.

105. Oosthuizen PP, Emsley RA, Maritz JS, et al. Incidence of tardive dyskinesia in first-episode psychosis patients treated with low-dose haloperidol. J Clin Psychiatry 2003;64(9):1075–80.

106. Jeste DV. Tardive dyskinesia in older patients. J Clin Psychiatry 2000;61(Suppl 4):27–32.

107. Miller DD, McEvoy JP, Davis SM, et al. Clinical correlates of tardive dyskinesia in schizophrenia: baseline data from the CATIE schizophrenia trial. Schizophr Res 2005;80(1):33–43.

108. Lv Z, Rong B, Tong X, et al. The association between COMT Val158Met gene polymorphism and antipsychotic-induced tardive dyskinesia risk. Int J Neurosci 2015;1–7.

109. Zai CC, Tiwari AK, Mazzoco M, et al. Association study of the vesicular monoamine transporter gene SLC18A2 with tardive dyskinesia. J Psychiatr Res 2013;47(11):1760–5.

110. Tsai HT, Caroff SN, Miller DD, et al. A candidate gene study of tardive dyskinesia in the CATIE schizophrenia trial. Am J Med Genet B Neuropsychiatr Genet 2009;153B(1):336–40.

111. Aberg K, Adkins DE, Bukszar J, et al. Genomewide association study of movement-related adverse antipsychotic effects. Biol Psychiatry 2010;67(3):279–82.

112. Beasley CM, Dellva MA, Tamura RN, et al. Randomised double-blind comparison of the incidence of tardive dyskinesia in patients with schizophrenia during long-term treatment with olanzapine or haloperidol. Br J Psychiatry 1999;174:23–30.

113. Jeste DV, Lacro JP, Bailey A, et al. Lower incidence of tardive dyskinesia with risperidone compared with haloperidol in older patients. J Am Geriatr Soc 1999;47(6):716–9.

114. Kane JM. Tardive dyskinesia circa 2006. Am J Psychiatry 2006;163(8):1316–8.

115. Kane JM, Woerner MG, Pollack S, et al. Does clozapine cause tardive dyskinesia? J Clin Psychiatry 1993;54(9):327–30.

116. Lieberman JA, Saltz BL, Johns CA, et al. The effects of clozapine on tardive dyskinesia. Br J Psychiatry 1991;158:503–10.

117. Jeste DV, Lohr JB, Clark K, et al. Pharmacological treatments of tardive dyskinesia in the 1980s. J Clin Psychopharmacol 1988;8(4 Suppl):38S–48S.

118. Bhidayasiri R, Fahn S, Weiner WJ, et al. Evidence-based guideline: treatment of tardive syndromes: report of the Guideline Development Subcommittee of the American Academy of Neurology. Neurology 2013;81(5):463–9.

119. Lockwood JT, Remington G. Emerging drugs for antipsychotic-induced tardive dyskinesia: investigational drugs in phase II and phase III clinical trials. Expert Opin Emerg Drugs 2015;20(3):407–21.
120. Jankovic J, Clarence-Smith K. Tetrabenazine for the treatment of chorea and other hyperkinetic movement disorders. Expert Rev Neurother 2011;11(11): 1509–23.
121. O'Brien CF, Jimenez R, Hauser RA, et al. NBI-98854, a selective monoamine transport inhibitor for the treatment of tardive dyskinesia: a randomized, double-blind, placebo-controlled study. Mov Disord 2015;30(12):1681–7.
122. Pappa S, Tsouli S, Apostolou G, et al. Effects of amantadine on tardive dyskinesia: a randomized, double-blind, placebo-controlled study. Clin Neuropharmacol 2010;33(6):271–5.
123. Miller R, Chouinard G. Loss of striatal cholinergic neurons as a basis for tardive and L-dopa-induced dyskinesias, neuroleptic-induced supersensitivity psychosis and refractory schizophrenia. Biol Psychiatry 1993;34(10):713–38.
124. Caroff SN, Campbell EC, Havey J, et al. Treatment of tardive dyskinesia with donepezil: a pilot study. J Clin Psychiatry 2001;62(10):772–5.
125. Caroff SN, Walker P, Campbell C, et al. Treatment of tardive dyskinesia with galantamine: a randomized controlled crossover trial. J Clin Psychiatry 2007; 68(3):410–5.
126. Quik M, Bordia T, Zhang D, et al. Nicotine and nicotinic receptor drugs: potential for Parkinson's disease and drug-induced movement disorders. Int Rev Neurobiol 2015;124:247–71.
127. Di Paolo T, Gregoire L, Feuerbach D, et al. AQW051, a novel and selective nicotinic acetylcholine receptor alpha7 partial agonist, reduces L-dopa-induced dyskinesias and extends the duration of L-Dopa effects in parkinsonian monkeys. Parkinsonism Relat Disord 2014;20(11):1119–23.
128. Shen W, Plotkin JL, Francardo V, et al. M4 muscarinic receptor signaling ameliorates striatal plasticity deficits in models of L-DOPA-induced dyskinesia. Neuron 2015;88(4):762–73.

Serotonin Reuptake Inhibitors and Risk of Abnormal Bleeding

Chittaranjan Andrade, MD[a],*, Eesha Sharma, MD[b]

KEYWORDS

- Antidepressant • Serotonin reuptake inhibitor • Selective serotonin reuptake inhibitor
- Bleeding • Postpartum hemorrhage • Intracranial hemorrhage
- Nonsteroidal anti-inflammatory drugs • Antiplatelet drugs

KEY POINTS

- Antidepressants with potent serotonin reuptake inhibitor (SRI) activity increase the risk of bleeding through different mechanisms.
- The upper gastrointestinal (GI) tract is the commonest site of SRI-related abnormal bleeding.
- The risk of SRI-related upper GI bleeding is raised by concurrent treatment with nonsteroidal anti-inflammatory drugs, antiplatelet drugs, and anticoagulant drugs; the risk is lowered by acid-suppressing drugs.
- SRIs may also increase the risk of intracranial bleeding, perioperative bleeding, postpartum bleeding, and bleeding at various sites in patients with liver disease.
- Patients are at risk of SRI-related abnormal bleeding primarily during the period of actual use.

Serotonin reuptake inhibitor (SRI) drugs (**Box 1**), which include the selective serotonin reuptake inhibitors (SSRIs) and antidepressants such as clomipramine and venlafaxine, are extensively prescribed in psychiatry for short- and long-term use across a range of diagnoses. This article updates an earlier review[1] on bleeding as an adverse effect (AE) of SRI treatment.[1] Although most of the research addresses SSRI use, the findings are conceptually applicable to all potent SRIs.

Funding: None.
Conflict of Interest: None related to the subject of this article.
[a] Department of Psychopharmacology, National Institute of Mental Health and Neurosciences, Bangalore 560 029, India; [b] Department of Psychiatry, King George's Medical University, Lucknow 226 003, India
* Corresponding author.
E-mail address: andradec@gmail.com

Box 1
Important serotonin-reuptake inhibitor drugs

Selective serotonin reuptake inhibitors:

Fluoxetine, sertraline, paroxetine, fluvoxamine, citalopram, escitalopram

Other potent serotonin reuptake inhibitors:

Clomipramine, venlafaxine, vilazodone

MECHANISMS OF ABNORMAL BLEEDING ASSOCIATED WITH SEROTONIN REUPTAKE INHIBITORS

Platelets release serotonin in response to vascular injury; this triggers vasoconstriction and platelet aggregation, resulting in hemostasis. SRIs inhibit uptake of serotonin into platelets much as they inhibit reuptake of serotonin into presynaptic neurons; because platelets do not synthesize serotonin, the SRI effect results in serotonin depletion in platelets, and hence, reduced efficiency of hemostasis.[1]

SSRIs also increase gastric acidity, which may explain why most of the literature on SSRI-related bleeding addresses upper gastrointestinal (GI) bleeds.[1] In this context, a population-based case-control study found that SSRI users (compared with nonusers) had odds of 1.5 (95% confidence interval [CI], 1.18–1.90) of uncomplicated peptic ulcers.[2]

SSRIs may reduce platelet/endothelial activation beyond that associated with concurrent antiplatelet drugs such as aspirin and clopidogrel.[3,4] Other indirect platelet-related mechanisms include interaction with the glycogen IIb/IIIa surface receptor involved in platelet activation.[5] Also, long-term treatment with sertraline upregulates the expression of glycogen synthase kinase 3-β(GSK3B) on platelets[6]; GSK3B acts as a negative regulator of platelet function and thrombosis and might contribute to bleeding risk with SRI use.

Cardiovascular and cerebrovascular benefits associated with these mechanisms are reviewed elsewhere.[7] The timelines for bleeding risks are presented in **Boxes 2** and **3**.[8]

SITES OF ABNORMAL BLEEDING

SRI-related bleeding has been reported at several important sites. These sites are listed in **Box 4**. Stray reports describe bleeding at other sites[9–17]; in this context, underreporting may be a problem because patients, caregivers, and physicians may not suspect a connection between the bleeding and the SRI. In support of such case reports, which by themselves do not constitute evidence, one study[18] reported that in patients taking SSRIs and coumarins, there was an increased risk of bleeding from non-GI sites such as the eye, nose, joints, skin, respiratory tract, uterus, or sites of surgical procedure (odds ratio [OR] = 1.7; 95% CI, 1.1 to 2.5).

EVIDENCE OF ABNORMAL BLEEDING: GENERAL ISSUES

Meta-analyses of observational studies have found ORs of 1.5 to 1.6 for risk of upper GI bleeding with SRIs[19,20] (**Box 5**). Meta-analysis also suggests SSRI-related increased risk of intracranial hemorrhage (relative risk [RR] = 1.51; 95% CI, 1.26–1.81) and intracerebral hemorrhage (RR = 1.42; 95% CI, 1.23–1.65),[21,22] and

Box 2
Risk period for the occurrence of serotonin reuptake inhibitor–related abnormal bleeding

Probable time of onset of bleeding risk with SRIs

1. From the time that serotonin reuptake inhibition becomes clinically significant, such as when the drug reaches steady state levels after dose initiation, or even earlier. However, platelet serotonin levels may need to fall below a certain threshold for impaired platelet activity to become clinically significant; this may take weeks.[1]

2. From the time that the drug increases gastric acidity. However, a mucosal lesion must exist for bleeding to occur. Mucosal ulceration and bleeding will not occur in everybody, and certainly not immediately after starting SSRI treatment even if these drugs do increase gastric acidity.

Examples of supporting studies

1. Dall and colleagues[29] found that the risk of SSRI-related GI bleeding was highest during the initial weeks of treatment.

2. Loke and colleagues[31] analyzed 101 spontaneous reports and found that upper GI bleeding occurred after a median of 25 weeks of SSRI treatment. About 67% of these patients were also receiving NSAIDs.

Conclusions and comments

1. Some persons may already be at risk at the time of SRI initiation, and these persons may experience early bleeds.

2. Persons who are not at risk may take a variable duration of time to develop abnormality such as a mucosal ulceration, or to add to their risk factors such as with addition of NSAID or anticoagulant drugs to the prescription. Therefore, time to bleeding may be very variable in such persons.

3. Persons who suffer GI discomfort after SSRI initiation, and hence those who might be vulnerable to GI bleeds as an AE, may stop treatment. That is, they may self-select themselves out of longer-term treatment, eliminating their risk of a GI bleed.

4. Effectively, patients are at risk all through the period of treatment.

Box 3
End of risk period for the occurrence of serotonin reuptake inhibitor–related abnormal bleeding

Probable end of risk period for abnormal bleeding with SRIs

The risk of SRI-related abnormal bleeding is likely to end after increased gastric acidity and serotonin reuptake inhibition are no longer clinically significant, such as when the drug is washed out of the body after SRI discontinuation.

Example of supporting study

Dalton and colleagues[8] found that the risk of SSRI-related abnormal bleeding was increased only during the period that the SSRIs were taken. Many other studies have similarly found that patients are at risk of SRI-related abnormal bleeding when they are current users, not when they are recent users or past users. This is noted at various points in the text.

Implications

Patients who require elective surgery can taper and temporarily stop their SRI medication (if their clinical state permits it) so that their risk of perioperative bleeding is reduced.

Box 4

Sites, nature, and contexts of serotonin reuptake inhibitor–related abnormal bleeding

Upper gastrointestinal bleeding

Intracranial bleeding

Postpartum hemorrhage

Perioperative bleeding

Bleeding associated with liver disease

Miscellaneous reports: ecchymoses; bleeding from the gums; epistaxis; subconjunctival hemorrhage; vaginal bleeding; epidural hematoma; hemorrhagic patellar bursitis; bleeding into joints; retrobulbar hematoma

---

increased need for perioperative blood transfusions (OR = 1.19; 95% CI, 1.09–1.30).[23]

Concurrent use of nonsteroidal anti-inflammatory drugs (NSAIDs) and antiplatelet drugs increase the risk of bleeding several fold, with ORs ranging from 4 to 10[19,20]; use of proton pump inhibitors (PPIs) and acid suppressants reduce this risk, specifically for GI bleeding.

Importantly, the ability of a study to detect SSRI-related upper GI bleeding depends not only on sample size but also on duration of observation (see **Box 2**).

ANTIDEPRESSANTS THAT INCREASE THE RISK OF ABNORMAL BLEEDING

Almost without exception, studies on antidepressant-related abnormal bleeding implicate SRIs. In a meta-analysis, paroxetine, fluoxetine, fluvoxamine, sertraline, and venlafaxine were found to carry comparable risks of bleeding (ORs, 1.3–1.7), whereas higher odds were associated with citalopram and escitalopram (OR > 2).[20]

In a study that examined interactions, citalopram (OR = 1.73; 95% CI, 1.25–2.38), fluoxetine (OR = 1.63; 95% CI, 1.11–2.38), paroxetine (OR = 1.64; 95% CI, 1.27–2.12), amitriptyline (OR = 1.47; 95% CI, 1.02–2.11), and even mirtazapine (OR = 1.75; 95% CI, 1.30–2.35) increased the risk of GI bleeding comparably in warfarin users.[24]

Box 5

Summary of findings from meta-analysis on use of selective serotonin reuptake inhibitors and risk of upper gastrointestinal bleeding

Aim: To determine whether use of SSRIs affects the risk of upper gastrointestinal bleed (UGIB).

Studies included: 6 cohort and 16 case-control studies with >1,073,000 individuals.

Major findings:
  i. The odds of developing UGIB were 1.55-fold higher (95% CI, 1.35–1.78) in SSRI users.
  ii. A higher risk of UGIB was found with concurrent use of SSRIs and NSAIDs (OR = 10.90; 95% CI, 7.33–16.21) or antiplatelet drugs (OR = 5.00; 95% CI, 3.49–7.17).
  iii. The risk was increased with concurrent use of all 3 drugs (OR = 9.13; 95% CI, 1.12–74.77).
  iv. The risk was eliminated by use of acid-suppressing drugs (OR = 0.81; 95% CI, 0.43–1.53)

Data from Jiang HY, Chen HZ, Hu XJ, et al. Use of selective serotonin reuptake inhibitors and risk of upper gastrointestinal bleeding: a systematic review and meta-analysis. Clin Gastroenterol Hepatol 2015;13(1):42–50.e3.

In some studies, the potency of serotonin reuptake inhibition has been reported to affect the risk of GI bleeding, with paroxetine, fluoxetine, sertraline, and clomipramine linked to higher risks.[25,26] In an incident user cohort study of more than 35,000 SRI-treated depressed individuals, high-affinity SRIs were associated with a greater risk of GI and other bleeding events than low-affinity SRIs.[27]

MAGNITUDE OF RISK

A meta-analysis of 15 case-control and 4 cohort studies of SSRI use for any indication found a number needed to harm (NNH) of 3177 per year in a low-risk population (with a low base rate of GI bleeding, ie, no prior history of GI bleed, NSAID use, or anticoagulant use; no history of peptic ulcer disease; and taking into consideration age and gender), and an NNH of 881 in a high-risk population (with a high base rate of GI bleeding, ie, with a prior history of GI bleed, NSAID use, or anticoagulant use).[19] Another meta-analysis reported a higher risk (NNH = 791).[20]

The risk is increased when SRIs are administered along with antiplatelet drugs or NSAIDs, and the risk is highest (NNH = 53) when SRIs, antiplatelet drugs, and NSAIDs are used together.[20] The NNH for postpartum hemorrhage (PPH) was found to be 80 for women on serotonergic antidepressants and 97 for women on nonserotonergic antidepressants.[28] Thus, the magnitude of risk depends on the population treated and the circumstances associated with SRI use.

NONSTEROIDAL ANTI-INFLAMMATORY DRUGS AND THE RISK OF SEROTONIN REUPTAKE INHIBITOR–RELATED BLEEDING

NSAIDs, which themselves increase the risk of upper GI bleeds, magnify the risk of SRI-related bleeding. A large, population-based case-control study[29] found that the ORs for GI bleeding increased from 1.70 (95% CI, 1.46–1.92) in current SSRI users to 8.00 (95% CI, 4.8–13.0) with concurrent use of SSRIs and NSAIDs to 28.0 (95% CI, 7.6–103.0) with concurrent use of SSRIs, NSAIDs, and aspirin. Not all population-based studies find additional risk with the combination.[30] Nevertheless, a recent meta-analysis[19] found that the OR for upper GI bleeding was 1.6 (95% CI, 1.44–1.92) in SSRI users and 4.25 (95% CI, 2.82–6.42) in those who used SSRIs and NSAIDs together. An earlier meta-analysis, while identifying a 6 times higher OR for treatment with the combination, found that the absolute risk was low.[31]

Interestingly, some studies suggest that the risk of bleeding with the SRI-NSAID combination is greater than the additive risk of the individual drugs.[32]

Meta-analysis also indicates that the combination of duloxetine and NSAIDs carries a higher bleeding risk than duloxetine alone, and that the risk with duloxetine and NSAIDs is not very different from that with placebo and NSAIDs.[33] This finding suggests that duloxetine, which is less serotonergic than the SRIs, may not significantly increase the risk of abnormal bleeding.

Physicians who augment SRIs with celecoxib or aspirin with a view to increasing antidepressant action should be aware of the heightened bleeding risk.[34]

ANTIPLATELET/ANTICOAGULANT DRUGS AND THE RISK OF SEROTONIN REUPTAKE INHIBITOR–RELATED BLEEDING

A large case control study[24] found that warfarin users had an increased risk of GI bleeding after initiation of citalopram, fluoxetine, paroxetine, amitriptyline, or mirtazapine. These findings are supported by several population- and hospital-based studies that suggest that the risk of bleeding increases by at least 2 to 3 times when SRIs are combined with antiplatelet/anticoagulant drugs.[1] However, some studies report that aspirin, warfarin, and clopidogrel do not increase risks when combined with SSRIs or tricyclic antidepressants (TCAs).[35,36] A qualitative appraisal suggests that SSRIs probably do increase the risk of abnormal bleeding associated with antiplatelet/anticoagulant drugs, especially aspirin, including low dose aspirin as used in cardiovascular prophylaxis.[37]

PROTON PUMP INHIBITORS AND THE RISK OF SEROTONIN REUPTAKE INHIBITOR–RELATED BLEEDING

As earlier discussed, SRIs may increase gastric acid production, peptic ulceration, and hence upper GI bleeds. Logically, then, PPIs should attenuate this bleeding risk. Studies have indeed found this to be the case.[29,30] As an example, a case-control study of 1321 patients with upper GI bleeding and 10,000 matched controls[38] found that the synergistic effect of SSRIs and NSAIDs on bleeding risk was magnified among those not using acid-suppressing agents (OR = 9.1; 95% CI, 4.8–17.3) but was not significant among users of acid-suppressing agents (OR = 1.3; 95% CI, 0.5–3.3). Similarly, the association between SSRIs and bleeding was enhanced by the concurrent use of antiplatelet agents in nonusers of acid-suppressing agents (OR = 4.7; 95% CI, 2.6–8.3) but was not significant among users of acid-suppressing agents (OR = 0.8; 95% CI, 0.3–2.5).

INTRACRANIAL BLEEDING

Some (but not all) studies suggest that SRIs increase intracranial bleeding (**Boxes 6** and **7**[39–42]). However, a meta-analysis of 52 RCTs with a pooled sample of greater than 4000 subjects suggested that, in stroke survivors, SSRI use reduced dependence, disability, neurologic impairment, depression, and anxiety without significantly increasing bleeding risk.[43] This finding indicates that, even if SRIs do increase the risk of intracranial bleeding, the risk is likely to be small and clinically insignificant.

ABNORMAL BLEEDING ASSOCIATED WITH SURGICAL PROCEDURES

A retrospective study of more than 530,000 adults who underwent major surgery showed that SSRI use slightly but significantly raised the odds of later bleeding (OR = 1.09; 95% CI, 1.04–1.15).[44] However, analysis of patient/SSRI factors contributing to risk could not be studied.

A meta-analysis of 8 cohort studies with 79,976 SRI users and 485,336 non-antidepressant users[23] (**Box 8**) showed that SRI use slightly but significantly increased

---

Box 6
Examples of studies that suggest that selective serotonin reuptake inhibitors increase intracranial bleeding

A meta-analysis of controlled observational studies[21] found that both intracranial (RR = 1.51; 95% CI, 1.26–1.81) and intracerebral (RR = 1.42; 95% CI, 1.23–1.65) hemorrhage were associated with SSRI use. The risk was greater when SSRIs were used in combination with anticoagulants than when used alone.

Another meta-analysis of case-control and cohort studies[22] found that SSRIs were associated with an increased risk of ischemic (OR = 1.48; 95% CI, 1.08–2.02) as well as hemorrhagic (OR = 1.32; 95% CI, 1.02–1.71) stroke.

Box 7
Examples of studies that suggest that selective serotonin reuptake inhibitors do not increase intracranial bleeding

A systematic review of the 1966 to 2003 literature[38] noted that 2 case-control studies failed to show an association between SSRI use and intracranial hemorrhage. None of 16 studies of SSRI treatment in poststroke patients recorded significant cerebrovascular adverse reactions.

A case-control study[39] found that SSRI use was not associated with an increased risk of intracerebral or subarachnoid hemorrhage, nor did SSRIs potentiate the risk of these events in association with warfarin or antiplatelets agents. The study, however, was not adequately powered to identify a less than 60% elevation of risk.

A large nested case-control study found no association between SSRI or TCA use and hemorrhagic stroke,[40] regardless of a prior history of cerebrovascular events.

In ischemic stroke survivors,[41] SSRIs did not increase the risk of intracranial bleeding (HR = 1.14; 95% CI, 0.62–2.12) but did increase the risk of other major bleeding events (HR = 1.33; 95% CI, 1.14–1.55).

---

the need for transfusion (OR = 1.19; 95% CI, 1.09–1.30) but not need for reoperation for a bleeding event. In patients undergoing coronary artery bypass graft (CABG) surgery there was no greater need for transfusion.

The risk of SRI-related perioperative bleeding depends on current use. For example, in women operated on for breast cancer,[45] the risk of reoperation for postoperative bleeding was increased in current SSRI users (RR = 2.3; 95% CI, 1.4–3.9) compared with never/past users.

Examples of studies on site and type of surgery are presented in **Box 9**.[46–52] The paucity of research on SRI-related abnormal surgical and dental bleeding is surprising, given the extent of study of GI bleeding. Possible reasons are considered in **Box 10**.[1]

Box 8
Summary of findings from meta-analysis on preoperative use of serotonergic antidepressants and risk of bleeding

Aim: To evaluate the association between preoperative serotonergic antidepressants (SAD) use and the risk of bleeding/mortality in patients undergoing surgery.

Studies included: 8 cohort studies with a pooled sample size of 79,976 SAD users and 485,336 non-antidepressant users.

Major findings:
 i. SAD use was not associated with increased requirement of reoperation for bleeding event (OR = 1.48; 95% CI, 0.84–2.62).
 ii. SAD use was associated with an increased requirement of transfusion (OR = 1.19; 95% CI, 1.09–1.30).
 iii. SAD use was associated with a substantial increase in mortality (OR = 1.53; 95% CI, 1.15–2.04) in patients undergoing CABG surgery but not in the overall population (OR = 1.1; 95% CI, 0.99–1.22).

Thus, an increased requirement of transfusion was found with preoperative SAD use; however, the divergence between CABG and other surgical groups needs to be examined in future research.

Data from Singh I, Achuthan S, Chakrabarti A, et al. Influence of pre-operative use of serotonergic antidepressants (SADs) on the risk of bleeding in patients undergoing different surgical interventions: a meta-analysis. Pharmacoepidemiol Drug Saf 2015;24(3):237–45.

Box 9

Serotonin reuptake inhibitors use and perioperative bleeding based on type and site of surgery

Bleeding risk has been found to be elevated in patients undergoing breast cosmetic surgery,[45] orthopedic surgery,[46,47] and spinal surgery.[48]

Studies on patients who underwent facelift surgery,[49] CABG surgery,[36,50] and oral or dental procedures[51] did not show this elevated risk.

ABNORMAL BLEEDING IN WOMEN

There are stray reports of SSRI-related vaginal bleeding[1] and one subgroup analysis which suggests that SRI potency is unrelated to vaginal bleeding risk in women with vaginal bleeding disorders.[25]

There is no published evidence to indicate that SRIs increase menstrual flow. A large, multicenter, case-control study reported a significantly higher prevalence of menstrual disorders in women on antidepressants such as paroxetine, venlafaxine, sertraline and mirtazapine.[53] This study reported the incidence of antidepressant-related menstruation disorders at 14.5%. However, a meta-analysis[54] that looked at the efficacy of antidepressants in the treatment of premenstrual syndrome, and that reported common AEs, did not report menstrual disturbance as one of the AEs.

An early case-control study found no association between SSRI use and PPH.[55] A subsequent large cohort study[28] found that all antidepressant classes increased the risk of PPH with an NNH of 80 for current exposure to SRIs, and 97 for non-SRIs. Another large cohort study[56] found no association between any class of antidepressant and vaginal bleeding during early or mid pregnancy, or PPH after vaginal or cesarean delivery. Only one hospital-based cohort study[57] found an SSRI-related increased risk of PPH after vaginal, nonsurgical delivery, relative to women who did not use SSRIs (OR = 2.6; 95% CI, 2.0–3.5). Blood loss was also higher in SSRI users relative to nonusers (484 vs 398 mL, respectively). However, there were no data on risks associated with non-SSRI use, or with untreated depression. A reasonable conclusion is that the risk of PPH, if increased, is related to either depression or to antidepressant use, regardless of antidepressant class, and so no especial proscription of SRIs is warranted on this count.

The risk of different kinds of bleeding in SRI-treated women definitely requires better study; for the present, however, the data are not alarming.

Box 10

Possible reasons why literature is limited on serotonin reuptake inhibitor–related abnormal surgical and dental bleeding

Nonessential medications are usually stopped before elective surgery. Platelet function may recover as SRI levels fall, leading to improved hemostasis.

It is difficult to accurately quantify and compare blood loss during and after surgery between SRI-exposed and unexposed groups.

Possibly because of lack of awareness, patients may not report, and dental surgeons may not ask about, use of SRIs at the time of dental procedures; so, excessive dental bleeding may be attributed to idiosyncrasy.

In patients undergoing CABG surgery, concurrent antiplatelet treatments may mask SRI-related risks.

Box 11

Risk factors for serotonin reuptake inhibitor–related abnormal bleeding

Old age

Concurrent treatment with NSAIDs, antiplatelet drugs, anticoagulants

Potential bleeding risk due to any cause, including bleeding disorders, chronic liver disease

Existing bleeding risk due to any cause, including acid peptic disease

Expected bleeding risk due to any cause, including obstetric, dental, or surgical events

Note: At present, there is no evidence that SRIs increase menstrual bleeding.

ABNORMAL BLEEDING ASSOCIATED WITH LIVER DISEASE

Hemostatic function may be compromised in liver disease. A small (n = 303), retrospective study found that SSRIs did not increase the risk of bleeding in hepatitis C patients treated with interferon.[58] A systematic review[59] of SSRI use in hepatitis C patients with cirrhosis and portal hypertension and/or hepatic failure identified 6 retrospective studies and 18 case reports of bleeding in 37 patients. A possible association between SSRI treatment and fatal GI bleeding was described in an additional patient. Bleeding events in 19 of 24 patients seemed closely associated with the use of SSRIs. The investigators suggested that aspirin or NSAIDs combined with SSRIs (prescribed for interferon-induced depression) might increase the risk of bleeding.

MANAGEMENT

SRI-induced hemostatic impairments may not be detectable by conventional laboratory methods; platelet aggregation tests are required to identify them but are not routinely done. SRI-related abnormal bleeding is uncommon; nevertheless, SRIs should be prescribed with caution, if indicated, in patients at risk (**Box 11**). Patients on an SRI should be told that, for pain, whenever possible they should take acetaminophen instead of aspirin.[60] Patients should be monitored for early signs of an increased tendency to bleed, which may include increased bruising and longer bleeding time after any injury, including phlebotomy, dental flossing, and shaving.[60]

Box 12

Examples of antidepressants that are unlikely to increase bleeding risks

Mirtazapine

Bupropion

Reboxetine

Agomelatine

Tianeptine

Monoamine oxidase inhibitors

Nutritional supplements, including L-methylfolate, S-adenosylmethionine, N-acetylcysteine

Unorthodox treatments, including low-dose amisulpride, pramipexole, ketamine

Note: These antidepressants have negligible or no SRI property.

> **Box 13**
> **Questions to be addressed in future research**
>
> Do specific patient characteristics increase the risk of abnormal bleeding with SRIs?
>
> Does the risk of abnormal bleeding increase with increasing potency of serotonin reuptake inhibition?
>
> Is the risk of abnormal bleeding different across different drugs?
>
> Is the risk of abnormal GI bleeding less with drugs that have potentially mitigating actions, such as anticholinergic action with clomipramine and paroxetine?
>
> Is the risk of abnormal bleeding dose-dependent?
>
> Does the experience of GI discomfort at the time of SRI initiation predict a later risk of abnormal GI bleeding?
>
> Is testing stools for occult blood a clinically useful method to screen for SRI-related GI bleeding?
>
> Is the risk of menstrual and postpartum bleeding increased by SRIs?

PPIs can attenuate GI bleeding risks in patients receiving SRIs prescribed alone or in combination with drugs that increase the bleeding risk; alternately, non-SRI antidepressants may be considered in such situations (**Box 12**). Stools should be periodically tested for occult blood in patients at risk of SRI-related GI bleeding. If clinically permissible, SRIs can be tapered and withdrawn before elective surgery and recommenced afterwards.

In the final reckoning, the benefits of SRI-related antiplatelet (and related) action[7] should be weighed against the risks of SRI-related abnormal bleeding. Further issues related to management and directions for future research (**Box 13**) are discussed elsewhere.[1]

REFERENCES

1. Andrade C, Sandarsh S, Chethan KB, et al. Serotonin reuptake inhibitor antidepressants and abnormal bleeding: a review for clinicians and a reconsideration of mechanisms. J Clin Psychiatry 2010;71(12):1565–75.
2. Dall M, Schaffalitzky de Muckadell OB, Lassen AT, et al. There is an association between selective serotonin reuptake inhibitor use and uncomplicated peptic ulcers: a population-based case-control study. Aliment Pharmacol Ther 2010; 32(11–12):1383–91.
3. Serebruany VL, Glassman AH, Malinin AI, et al. Selective serotonin reuptake inhibitors yield additional antiplatelet protection in patients with congestive heart failure treated with antecedent aspirin. Eur J Heart Fail 2003;5(4):517–21.
4. Serebruany VL, Glassman AH, Malinin AI, et al. Platelet/endothelial biomarkers in depressed patients treated with the selective serotonin reuptake inhibitor sertraline after acute coronary events: the Sertraline AntiDepressant Heart Attack Randomized Trial (SADHART) Platelet Substudy. Circulation 2003;108(8):939–44.
5. Galan AM, Lopez-Vilchez I, Diaz-Ricart M, et al. Serotonergic mechanisms enhance platelet-mediated thrombogenicity. Thromb Haemost 2009;102(3): 511–9.
6. Joaquim HP, Talib LL, Forlenza OV, et al. Long-term sertraline treatment increases expression and decreases phosphorylation of glycogen synthase kinase-3B in platelets of patients with late-life major depression. J Psychiatr Res 2012;46(8): 1053–8.

7. Andrade C, Kumar CB, Surya S. Cardiovascular mechanisms of SSRI drugs and their benefits and risks in ischemic heart disease and heart failure. Int Clin Psychopharmacol 2013;28(3):145–55.
8. Dalton SO, Johansen C, Mellemkjaer L. Use of selective serotonin reuptake inhibitors and risk of upper gastrointestinal tract bleeding: a population-based cohort study. Arch Intern Med 2003;163(1):59–64.
9. Shen WW, Swartz CM, Calhoun JW. Is inhibition of nitric oxide synthase a mechanism for SSRI-induced bleeding? Psychosomatics 1999;40(3):268–9.
10. Lake MB, Birmaher B, Wassick S, et al. Bleeding and selective serotonin reuptake inhibitors in childhood and adolescence. J Child Adolesc Psychopharmacol 2000;10(1):35–8.
11. Mowla A, Dastgheib SA, Ebrahimi AA, et al. Nasal bleeding associated with fluoxetine and risperidone interaction: a case report. Pharmacopsychiatry 2009;42(5):204–5.
12. Sharma RC. Escitalopram-induced subconjunctival hemorrhage: a case report. Prim Psychiatr 2009;16:29–30.
13. Akbulut S, Yagmur Y, Gumus S, et al. Breast ecchymosis: unusual complication of an antidepressant agent. Int J Surg Case Rep 2014;5(3):129–30.
14. Kaya I, Kocas S, Suleyman F, et al. Vaginal bleeding in a preadolescent girl possibly related to sertraline. J Clin Psychopharmacol 2014;34(6):760–1.
15. Turkoglu S, Turkoglu G. Vaginal bleeding and hemorrhagic prepatellar bursitis in a preadolescent girl, possibly related to fluoxetine. J Child Adolesc Psychopharmacol 2015;25(2):186–7.
16. Sagar A, Hassan K. Drug interaction as cause of spontaneously resolving epidural spinal hematoma on warfarin therapy. J Neurosci Rural Pract 2010;1(1):39–42.
17. Van Cann EM, Koole R. Retrobulbar hematoma associated with selective serotonin reuptake inhibitor: a case report. Oral Surg Oral Med Oral Pathol Oral Radiol Endod 2009;108(4):e1–2.
18. Schalekamp T, Klungel OH, Souverein PC. Increased bleeding risk with concurrent use of selective serotonin reuptake inhibitors and coumarins. Arch Intern Med 2008;168(2):180–5.
19. Anglin R, Yuan Y, Moayyedi P, et al. Risk of upper gastrointestinal bleeding with selective serotonin reuptake inhibitors with or without concurrent nonsteroidal anti-inflammatory use: a systematic review and meta-analysis. Am J Gastroenterol 2014;109(6):811–9.
20. Jiang HY, Chen HZ, Hu XJ, et al. Use of selective serotonin reuptake inhibitors and risk of upper gastrointestinal bleeding: a systematic review and meta-analysis. Clin Gastroenterol Hepatol 2015;13(1):42–50.e3.
21. Hackam DG, Mrkobrada M. Selective serotonin reuptake inhibitors and brain hemorrhage: a meta-analysis. Neurology 2012;79(18):1862–5.
22. Shin D, Oh YH, Eom CS, et al. Use of selective serotonin reuptake inhibitors and risk of stroke: a systematic review and meta-analysis. J Neurol 2014;261(4):686–95.
23. Singh I, Achuthan S, Chakrabarti A, et al. Influence of pre-operative use of serotonergic antidepressants (SADs) on the risk of bleeding in patients undergoing different surgical interventions: a meta-analysis. Pharmacoepidemiol Drug Saf 2015;24(3):237–45.
24. Schelleman H, Brensinger CM, Bilker WB, et al. Antidepressant-warfarin interaction and associated gastrointestinal bleeding risk in a case-control study. PLoS One 2011;6(6):e21447.

25. Meijer WE, Heerdink ER, Nolen WA, et al. Association of risk of abnormal bleeding with degree of serotonin reuptake inhibition by antidepressants. Arch Intern Med 2004;164(21):2367–70.

26. van Walraven C, Mamdani MM, Wells PS, et al. Inhibition of serotonin reuptake by antidepressants and upper gastrointestinal bleeding in elderly patients: retrospective cohort study. BMJ 2001;323(7314):655–8.

27. Castro VM, Gallagher PJ, Clements CC, et al. Incident user cohort study of risk for gastrointestinal bleed and stroke in individuals with major depressive disorder treated with antidepressants. BMJ Open 2012;2(2):e000544.

28. Palmsten K, Hernández-Díaz S, Huybrechts KF, et al. Use of antidepressants near delivery and risk of postpartum hemorrhage: cohort study of low income women in the United States. BMJ 2013;347:f4877.

29. Dall M, Schaffalitzky de Muckadell OB, Lassen AT, et al. An association between selective serotonin reuptake inhibitor use and serious upper gastrointestinal bleeding. Clin Gastroenterol Hepatol 2009;7(12):1314–21.

30. Targownik LE, Bolton JM, Metge CJ, et al. Selective serotonin reuptake inhibitors are associated with a modest increase in the risk of upper gastrointestinal bleeding. Am J Gastroenterol 2009;104(6):1475–82.

31. Loke YK, Trivedi AN, Singh S. Meta-analysis: gastrointestinal bleeding due to interaction between selective serotonin uptake inhibitors and non-steroidal anti-inflammatory drugs. Aliment Pharmacol Ther 2008;27(1):31–40.

32. Mort JR, Aparasu RR, Baer RK. Interaction between selective serotonin reuptake inhibitors and nonsteroidal antiinflammatory drugs: review of the literature. Pharmacotherapy 2006;26(9):1307–13.

33. Perahia DG, Bangs ME, Zhang Q, et al. The risk of bleeding with duloxetine treatment in patients who use nonsteroidal anti-inflammatory drugs (NSAIDs): analysis of placebo-controlled trials and post-marketing adverse event reports. Drug Healthc Patient Saf 2013;5:211–9.

34. Andrade C. Antidepressant augmentation with anti-inflammatory agents. J Clin Psychiatry 2014;75(9):975–7.

35. Opatrny L, Delaney JA, Suissa S. Gastro-intestinal haemorrhage risks of selective serotonin receptor antagonist therapy: a new look. Br J Clin Pharmacol 2008; 66(1):76–81.

36. Kim DH, Daskalakis C, Whellan DJ, et al. Safety of selective serotonin reuptake inhibitor in adults undergoing coronary artery bypass grafting. Am J Cardiol 2009;103(10):1391–5.

37. Labos C, Dasgupta K, Nedjar H, et al. Risk of bleeding associated with combined use of selective serotonin reuptake inhibitors and antiplatelet therapy following acute myocardial infarction. CMAJ 2011;183(16):1835–43.

38. de Abajo FJ, Garcia-Rodriguez LA. Risk of upper gastrointestinal tract bleeding associated with selective serotonin reuptake inhibitors and venlafaxine therapy: interaction with nonsteroidal anti-inflammatory drugs and effect of acid-suppressing agents. Arch Gen Psychiatry 2008;65(7):795–803.

39. Ramasubbu R. Cerebrovascular effects of selective serotonin reuptake inhibitors: a systematic review. J Clin Psychiatry 2004;65(12):1642–53.

40. Kharofa J, Sekar P, Haverbusch M, et al. Selective serotonin reuptake inhibitors and risk of hemorrhagic stroke. Stroke 2007;38(11):3049–51.

41. Douglas I, Smeeth L, Irvine D. The use of antidepressants and the risk of haemorrhagic stroke: a nested case control study. Br J Clin Pharmacol 2011;71(1):116–20.

42. Mortensen JK, Larsson H, Johnsen SP, et al. Post stroke use of selective serotonin reuptake inhibitors and clinical outcome among patients with ischemic stroke: a nationwide propensity score-matched follow-up study. Stroke 2013;44(2):420–6.

43. Mead GE, Hsieh CF, Lee R, et al. Selective serotonin reuptake inhibitors (SSRIs) for stroke recovery. Cochrane Database Syst Rev 2012;(11):CD009286.

44. Auerbach AD, Vittinghoff E, Maselli J, et al. Perioperative use of selective serotonin reuptake inhibitors and risks for adverse outcomes of surgery. JAMA Intern Med 2013;173(12):1075–81.

45. Gartner R, Cronin-Fenton D, Hundborg HH, et al. Use of selective serotonin reuptake inhibitors and risk of re-operation due to post-surgical bleeding in breast cancer patients: a Danish population-based cohort study. BMC Surg 2010;10:3.

46. Basile FV, Basile AR, Basile VV. Use of selective serotonin reuptake inhibitors antidepressants and bleeding risk in breast cosmetic surgery. Aesthetic Plast Surg 2013;37(3):561–6.

47. Movig KL, Janssen MW, de Waal Malefijt J, et al. Relationship of serotonergic antidepressants and need for blood transfusion in orthopedic surgical patients. Arch Intern Med 2003;163(19):2354–8.

48. Schutte HJ, Jansen S, Schafroth MU, et al. SSRIs increase risk of blood transfusion in patients admitted for hip surgery. PLoS One 2014;9(5):e95906.

49. Sayadipour A, Mago R, Kepler CK, et al. Antidepressants and the risk of abnormal bleeding during spinal surgery: a case-control study. Eur Spine J 2012;21(10):2070–8.

50. Harirchian S, Zoumalan RA, Rosenberg DB. Antidepressants and bleeding risk after face-lift surgery. Arch Facial Plast Surg 2012;14(4):248–52.

51. Andreasen JJ, Riis A, Hjortdal VE, et al. Effect of selective serotonin reuptake inhibitors on requirement for allogeneic red blood cell transfusion following coronary artery bypass surgery. Am J Cardiovasc Drugs 2006;6(4):243–50.

52. Napenas JJ, Hong CH, Kempter E, et al. Selective serotonin reuptake inhibitors and oral bleeding complications after invasive dental treatment. Oral Surg Oral Med Oral Pathol Oral Radiol Endod 2011;112(4):463–7.

53. Uguz F, Sahingoz M, Kose SA, et al. Antidepressants and menstruation disorders in women: a cross-sectional study in three centers. Gen Hosp Psychiatry 2012; 34(5):529–33.

54. Marjoribanks J, Brown J, O'Brien PM, et al. Selective serotonin reuptake inhibitors for premenstrual syndrome. Cochrane Database Syst Rev 2013;(6):CD001396.

55. Salkeld E, Ferris LE, Juurlink DN. The risk of postpartum hemorrhage with selective serotonin reuptake inhibitors and other antidepressants. J Clin Psychopharmacol 2008;28(2):230–4.

56. Lupattelli A, Spigset O, Koren G, et al. Risk of vaginal bleeding and postpartum hemorrhage after use of antidepressants in pregnancy: a study from the Norwegian Mother and Child Cohort Study. J Clin Psychopharmacol 2014;34(1): 143–8.

57. Lindqvist PG, Nasiell J, Gustafsson LL, et al. Selective serotonin reuptake inhibitor use during pregnancy increases the risk of postpartum hemorrhage and anemia: a hospital-based cohort study. J Thromb Haemost 2014;12(12): 1986–92.

58. Martin KA, Krahn LE, Balan V, et al. Selective serotonin reuptake inhibitors in the context of hepatitis C infection: reexamining the risks of bleeding. J Clin Psychiatry 2007;68(7):1024–6.

59. Weinrieb RM, Auriacombe M, Lynch KG, et al. A critical review of selective serotonin reuptake inhibitor-associated bleeding: balancing the risk of treating hepatitis C-infected patients. J Clin Psychiatry 2003;64(12):1502–10.

60. Mago R, Mahajan R, Thase ME. Medically serious adverse effects of newer antidepressants. Curr Psychiatry Rep 2008;10(3):249–57.

Sexual Dysfunction Due to Psychotropic Medications

Anita H. Clayton, MD*, Andrew R. Alkis, MD, Nishant B. Parikh, MD,
Jennifer G. Votta, DO

KEYWORDS

- Sexual dysfunction • Antidepressant-induced sexual dysfunction
- Antipsychotic-induced sexual dysfunction
- Psychotropic-induced sexual dysfunction • Psychotropic adverse effects

KEY POINTS

- Sexual dysfunction (SD) associated with psychiatric illness or medication treatment involves neuroendocrine systems related to specific neuroanatomical structures, genetic factors, and psychological or social components.
- Serotonergic antidepressants, prolactin-inducing antipsychotic medications, and mood stabilizers or anticonvulsants that lower bioavailable testosterone are psychotropic medications most likely to negatively affect sexual functioning.
- Successful interventions that maintain therapeutic efficacy include adding an antidote, changing to a medication less likely to cause SD, and nonpharmacologic options.
- Taking a proactive approach to assessment and management of sexual functioning in psychiatric patients will enhance outcomes, adherence, and patient satisfaction.

INTRODUCTION

In modern medicine, psychotropic medicines are a mainstay on many patients' medication lists. Antidepressants are the most commonly prescribed medications in both Europe and the United States, with selective serotonin reuptake inhibitors (SSRIs) being at the forefront primarily due to safety and tolerability reasons.[1–3] This does not mean SSRIs are without their adverse effects and prescribers must have a firm knowledge of their pharmacodynamics, pharmacokinetics, and safety data. Many psychotropic medications have proven efficacy for various psychiatric indications; however, patients must be able to stay on medications for them to work.[4] It has been noted that as many as 20% of patients will discontinue treatment with an SSRI, with one-third of these patients doing so due to adverse reactions.[5] The SSRIs have many potential adverse effects; however, it can be argued that none are more disruptive than the

Department of Psychiatry and Neurobehavioral Sciences, University of Virginia, 1215 Lee Street, Charlottesville, VA 22903, USA
* Corresponding author. 2955 Ivy Road, Suite 210, Charlottesville, VA 22903.
E-mail address: ahc8v@virginia.edu

Psychiatr Clin N Am 39 (2016) 427–463
http://dx.doi.org/10.1016/j.psc.2016.04.006
0193-953X/16/$ – see front matter Published by Elsevier Inc.

psych.theclinics.com

sexual adverse effects. Sexual dysfunction (SD) as a result of SSRIs has been reported in the literature at a prevalence rate between 10% and 80%.[6,7] The wide variation is believed to be secondary to multiple factors, including age of the patient, comorbid medical illness (eg, cardiac disease, diabetes, vascular disease), and variable use of assessment tools (eg, Changes in Sexual Functioning Questionnaire [CSFQ], Arizona Sexual Experiences Scale [ASEX]). It is also important to note that only about 20% of patients spontaneously report their sexual adverse effects.[6]

One of the many difficulties in researching SD due to psychotropic medication is that mood, thought, and anxiety disorders can be associated with SD due to anhedonia, irritability, decreased concentration, and negative symptoms. In patients with major depressive disorder, the prevalence of pretreatment SD is estimated to range from 40% to 65%.[8] Decreased sleep, energy, and appetite can also lead to sequelae in the form of decreased vascular health. Other risk factors for SD (eg, smoking, alcohol consumption, and sexual trauma) are often more prevalent in individuals suffering from depression or other psychiatric comorbidities (eg, post-traumatic stress disorder).[9] Regardless of the cause, sexual functioning is strongly associated with quality of life. If dysfunction is present and occurring secondary to medication, this can serve to worsen a patient's depression or anxiety.[10–12]

BIOLOGY OF THE SEXUAL RESPONSE: NORMAL AND IN DEPRESSION

The human sexual response is mediated by various neurotransmitters (eg, dopamine, serotonin, acetylcholine, nitric oxide) and hormones (eg, testosterone) in specific brain structures (eg, hypothalamus, limbic system, cortex)[13–15] (**Fig. 1**). Traditionally, the stages of the sexual response cycle have been classified as desire, arousal, and orgasm.[14] The serotonergic system plays a largely inhibitory role on sexual desire, orgasm, and ejaculation with involvement of the hippocampus and amygdala.[16] However, serotonin's effects in the central nervous system are determined by the specific receptors activated. For example, 5- hydroxytryptamine (HT)-type 2 and 5-HT3 receptors inhibit sexual activity, whereas 5-HT1A receptors stimulate these functions.[16] Dopamine plays a central role through its involvement in the mesolimbic pathway and reward system. Dopaminergic activation of the nucleus accumbens and the

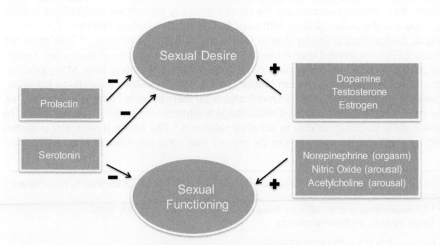

Fig. 1. Neurotransmitters and their effects on sexual functioning and sexual desire: increase (*plus sign*) and decrease (*minus sign*). (*Data from* Refs.[12,14,15])

medial preoptic hypothalamic region are essential to sexual motivation. Dopaminergic activation of the hypothalamic paraventricular nucleus is important to establishment of penile erections.[16] See later discussion for specifics on the sexual response cycle and how various psychotropic medications affect this cycle.

The sexual response cycle is negatively affected in individuals suffering from major depressive disorder, even before initiation of any psychotropic medication.[17] Men with depression have an increased incidence of reduced sexual interest or arousal (40% of unmedicated men) and reduced ability to reach orgasm or ejaculation (20% of unmedicated men).[18] Functional MRI (fMRI) of depressed women actively visualizing sexually stimulating imagery has shown less activation in certain brain regions (eg, middle occipital gyrus, middle temporal gyrus, inferior frontal gyrus, insula, hypothalamus, septal area, anterior cingulate gyrus, parahippocampal gyrus, thalamus, and amygdala) in comparison with women without depression.[19]

PATHOPHYSIOLOGY OF ADVERSE EFFECTS
Antidepressants and Antipsychotics

Sexuality is affected by psychological, environmental, and social factors, and a balance between these is essential for healthy sexual functioning. A mind-body model for sexual medicine has been presented that highlights the importance of assessing not only the physiologic aspects of SD but also the psychological.[13] The psychological aspects of SD can be addressed through psychotherapy, although it may require medication to combat the physiologic dysfunction.[20] The pathophysiology of SD remains an ongoing area of research. However, certain neurotransmitters and neurologic pathways have been implicated in not only the cause of antidepressant-associated SD but also SD due to other psychotropic medications (eg, atypical antipsychotics). Serotonin and dopamine seem to be strongly implicated in the process. Glutamate, nitric oxide, prolactin, and acetylcholine also seem to play a role.[15]

During the sexual desire phase in both men and women, plasma testosterone is necessary for desire or interest, influencing specific brain regions that are sensitive to internal and external sexual cues.[21] The blood level of testosterone is affected by prolactin because testosterone release is directly inhibited by prolactin. Medications that increase the levels of prolactin (eg, antipsychotics, tricyclic antidepressants [TCAs]), will indirectly suppress the level of testosterone.[8] Hyperprolactinemia also increases GABAergic activity and endogenous opioid levels, which both negatively affect libido and erection.[22] Prolactin levels are regulated by hypothalamic dopamine, which has a tonic inhibitory effect. Medications that suppress dopaminergic activity (eg, antipsychotics) will cause an indirect increase in prolactin due to a loss of this inhibition.[16] Men with Parkinson's disease treated with levodopa (a dopamine precursor) sometimes report an increase in sexual libido.[23] Furthermore, women with hyperprolactinemia treated with bromocriptine (a dopamine agonist) sometimes report a return of sexual interest.[8] In contrast to the effects of dopamine on prolactin, increased serotonin activity promotes the release of prolactin.[8]

During male erection or female excitation (eg, lubrication and vaginal swelling), the peripheral autonomic nervous system is highly involved, particularly the parasympathetic nervous system with contributions from the lumbar spinal cord. Acetylcholine is prominent in the process of parasympathetic activation and leads to vasodilation in the erectile tissues of the penis and clitoris, and in the lining of the vagina. Nitric oxide also plays a role in this process.[24] Norepinephrine can play an inhibitory role through its ability to inhibit erection by binding to peripheral alpha-1 receptors.[25] Atypical antipsychotics can lead to priapism through blockade of alpha-1 adrenergic receptors.[26] Of note, a relationship has been shown between stimulation of 5-HT2C receptors and erection in the male rat.[27]

Ejaculation is a process primarily mediated by the sympathetic nervous system with contributions from the sacral spinal cord. This sympathetic activation in men leads to contraction of the smooth muscle in the epididymis, vas deferens, and seminal vesicles, propelling the ejaculate into the posterior urethra. The only contribution from the parasympathetic nervous system in this process is through the excretion of seminal fluid from the wall of the seminal vesicles. Ejaculation occurs following propulsion of the seminal fluid from the urethra via contraction of the surrounding muscle.[8] Norepinephrine, serotonin, and prolactin regulate ejaculation.[24] In the male rat, it has been demonstrated that ejaculation is influenced by the 5-HTA1 receptor subtype.[28] Orgasm itself seems to have an association with oxytocin. Oxytocin release has been noted in men during orgasm.[29] Interestingly, release of oxytocin is inhibited by naloxone (an opioid receptor antagonist).[30] Given this, it has been postulated that oxytocin may be responsible for the pleasant sensations experienced during orgasm.[8]

The neuroanatomy of ejaculation seems to be linked to the hypothalamus, brainstem, and spinal cord. The medial preoptic area of the hypothalamus is associated with ejaculation.[8,31] The paragigantocellular reticular nucleus located in the brainstem inhibits ejaculation.[32] The so-called spinal ejaculation center located in the spinal cord is responsible for the sympathetic and parasympathetic contributions to the ejaculatory process previously described.[33,34]

Effects of antidepressants on the classic reward system have also been evaluated using fMRI. On fMRI, paroxetine has been shown to decrease activation in response to visual erotic stimuli in both the ventral tegmental area and the pregenual anterior cingulate cortex in comparison with bupropion and placebo.[13]

Mood Stabilizers

In interpreting the data evaluating a relationship between mood stabilizers and SD, it is important to keep in mind that most of the data comes from studies in epilepsy rather than mood disorders. This is important because epilepsy itself also seems to be associated with SD.[35]

At this time, there is not a great deal of data on lithium and SD, although there seems to be an association between them. A recently published review included 8 investigations looking at the effects of lithium on SD.[36] In 1 of these studies, 35 subjects with bipolar disorder or schizoaffective disorder currently taking lithium were evaluated. Eleven subjects (31.4%) reported SD. Of these, 23% reported reduced sexual thoughts, 20% reported erectile failure, and 14% reported erectile dysfunction. SD was not correlated with lithium level.[37] The mechanism of SD caused by lithium is currently not well understood.

Valproic acid is linked to an increase in testosterone and estrogen levels, which can in turn lead to hirsutism and polycystic ovarian syndrome in women and reduced testicular volume in men.[38,39] There have been cases of severely decreased libido and anorgasmia in women with bipolar disorder who are taking valproic acid. The cause was hypothesized to be secondary to increased serotonergic activity induced by valproate.[40] Valproic acid is also associated with decreased sex hormone-binding globulin (SHBG), which in turn can increase the level of free testosterone. This relationship is believed to be the cause of hyperandrogenism in individuals taking valproate.[41]

Carbamazepine is associated with increased production of SHBG, which can potentially lead to decreased free testosterone and hypogonadism.[42] There are some case reports that have implicated oxcarbazepine as contributing to anorgasmia and retrograde ejaculation. However, the mechanism for these adverse effects is unclear.[43–45] In contrast, there is an open-label study of men with partial epilepsy on oxcarbazepine that assessed SD. Of the participants, 79.4% (181 subjects) reported an improvement in sexual function after 3 months on oxcarbazepine.[46]

For both gabapentin and pregabalin, there are case reports of anorgasmia and erectile dysfunction. Gabapentin has also been associated with decreased libido and anejaculation, and pregabalin delayed ejaculation as evidenced by case reports.[47–51] It has been hypothesized that gabapentin-induced SD occurs secondary to a central inhibitory effect on neurotransmission, although there is no evidence currently supporting this hypothesis.[52]

Lamotrigine seems to have little effect on SHBG and is not believed to be associated with SD.[53,54]

Benzodiazepines

Little is known regarding SD related to benzodiazepine anxiolytics; however, several theories have been hypothesized. Some investigators have noted benzodiazepines to be associated with reduced desire, delay in reaching orgasm, and erectile dysfunction; whereas others maintain drugs such as lorazepam and clonazepam promote sexual desire and disinhibition, respectively.[52] Given that hyperprolactinemia can inhibit sexual functioning through an increase in GABAergic activity, it is possible that benzodiazepines may cause SD through their GABA agonist properties.

PHARMACOGENETICS OF SELECTIVE SEROTONIN REUPTAKE INHIBITOR–ASSOCIATED SEXUAL DYSFUNCTION

There is heterogeneity present in individuals who present with antidepressant-associated SD that has led to a burgeoning field looking at genetic risk factors in the development of these adverse effects. Over the last several years, researchers have looked at various genetic contributors for a potential role in antidepressant-associated SD.[55]

Two studies have reported a higher incidence of SD with paroxetine in persons who were cytochrome P450 2D6 poor metabolizers. One of these studies included men and women with depression, whereas the second also included individuals with anxiety.[56,57]

Citalopram, escitalopram, sertraline, and to a lesser extent fluoxetine and fluvoxamine are substrates for the cytochrome P450 2C19 isoenzyme. There are no studies yet validating this; however, it is thought polymorphisms encoding for this isoenzyme could play a role in SD.[55]

ABCB1 is a gene that encodes for a p-glycoprotein that is involved in maintenance of the blood-brain barrier. In 1 study, the ABCB1 1236 C allele gene product was noted to be associated with SD in women with depression currently taking citalopram, escitalopram, paroxetine, or sertraline. These SSRIs are substrates of various p-glycoproteins coded for by ABCB1 single nucleotide polymorphisms (SNPs). The women were compared with women taking fluoxetine, which is not a substrate of an ABCB1 p-glycoprotein.[58] In a different study, the ABCB1 2677 G allele was associated with lubrication issues and treatment-emergent orgasm disorders in women with bulimia nervosa taking paroxetine.[59]

SLC6A4 is a gene encoding for the serotonin transporter promoter region, which is the drug target for SSRIs. In theory, patients with higher expression of various polymorphisms of this genotype could have an exaggerated response to SSRIs, leading to up-regulation of postsynaptic receptors such as 5HT2A, a receptor acted on by both SSRIs and atypical antipsychotics.[55] The SLC6A4 5HTTLPR L/L polymorphism has been associated with SD based on the CSFQ in both men and women with depression who were being treated with citalopram, escitalopram, fluoxetine, paroxetine, or sertraline.[60] A lack of association between SLC6A4 5-HTTLPR and SD has been shown in men and women with major depressive disorder and depression treated with fluoxetine and escitalopram or nortriptyline, respectively.[61,62] The SLC6A4 STin2 polymorphism was also found to not be associated with SD in men and women with depression in this same subject population.[60] In men with lifelong premature ejaculation responsive to sertraline, the 5-HTTLPR L_A/L_A polymorphism and STin2 12/12 polymorphism were associated with increased intravaginal ejaculation latency time.[63] In contrast, when Dutch men who had lifelong premature ejaculation were treated with paroxetine, the 5-HTTLPR polymorphism was not associated with intravaginal ejaculatory latency time improvement.[64] In an alternative study, it was reported that men and women older than 60 years, with anxiety, and taking escitalopram displayed diminished sexual desire if they possessed the 5HTTLPR L allele.[65]

HTR2A is a gene encoding for the 5-HT2A receptor. It has been noted that men and women with depression treated with citalopram, escitalopram, fluoxetine, paroxetine, and sertraline who carry the HTR2A-1438 G/G genotype were more likely to have antidepressant-associated SD.[66] HTR1A is a gene encoding for the 5-HT1A receptor. Men and women older than 60 years with anxiety and taking escitalopram were more likely to have diminished sexual desire if they possessed the HTR1A rs6295 G allele genotype or HTR2A-1438 A allele.[65] A study looking at Han Chinese men with major depressive disorder taking either an SSRI or venlafaxine showed the HTR2A-1438 A/A genotype to be associated with SD.[67] A study looking at Malaysian women with major depressive disorder in remission taking fluoxetine, sertraline, fluvoxamine, or escitalopram did not, however, show an association between the HTR2A genotype and sexual desire disorder.[68]

GNB3 is a gene encoding for a g-protein secondary messenger of the 5-HT2A receptor. One study failed to demonstrate an increased association with SD in men and women with depression on citalopram, escitalopram, fluoxetine, paroxetine, or sertraline who possessed the GNB3 genotype.[66]

BDNF is a gene encoding for a precursor to brain derived neurotrophic factor. A study of Chinese men and women with major depressive disorder on fluoxetine noted an association between the BDNF Val6Met encoding allele and decreased sexual desire.[69]

GRIK2, GRIA3, and GRIA1 are polymorphisms of various subunits of glutamate receptors (AMPA-GRIA1 and GRIA3 and kainite GRIK2). Glutamate is believed to play a role in the pathophysiology of antidepressant-induced SD, although the exact role has not been defined. A study looking at white men and women with major depressive disorder taking citalopram found that individuals with the GRIA3 and GRIK2 polymorphisms were more likely to report decreased libido. Presence of GRIN3A polymorphism was associated with ability to achieve erection, whereas GRIA1 polymorphisms were associated with difficulty achieving orgasm.[70] In another study, men and women with depression taking citalopram, escitalopram, fluoxetine, paroxetine, or sertraline showed that the GRIK2, GRIA3, and GRIA1 candidate SNPs studied were not associated with total scores on the CSFQ. However, the GRIA1 SNP rs1994862 was associated with arousal dysfunction.[71]

In summation, there is a great deal of on-going research investigating pharmacogenetics affecting liver metabolism, the blood brain barrier, serotonin receptor subunits, neurotrophic factors, and glutamate receptor subunits. The available data on these areas of focus are summarized in **Table 1**.

MEDICATION-INDUCED SEXUAL DYSFUNCTION

Before reviewing the existing evidence related to SD associated with various classes of psychiatric medications, it may be helpful to make a comment regarding the quality and origin of these studies. First, no standardized definition for SD exists. SD can occur in any of the 3 phases of the sexual response cycle and often it is not clear what phases or specific adverse effects are being evaluated when patients are being asked about SD. SD can include but is not limited to decrease in or loss of sexual desire, difficulty with erections, priapism, dysorgasmia, anorgasmia, dyspareunia, spontaneous orgasm, ejaculation disorders (delayed, inhibited, retrograde, spontaneous, decreased volume), sexual disinhibition, and sexual satisfaction. The term libido is often used loosely in some reports and is often not precise enough to define the quality of dysfunction.

Although there are several psychometric rating scales for SD, each has different sensitivity for SD. Many studies do not use a validated scale at all, often because the original primary or secondary objectives of these studies were not to research SD. As a result, baseline SD is often not established before initiation of medication.

Additionally, cultural norms regarding sexual function differ, resulting in variances in willingness of patients to report and of doctors to inquire[72] about differences in expectations of what is normal sexual functioning. It has been shown that studies published after the year 2000 report a significantly higher percentage of drug-induced SD compared with studies before that year.[73] Health professionals may not accurately estimate how much of the level of SD is due to the psychiatric illness versus the medications. It is important to keep these factors in mind when reviewing the current evidence (**Fig. 2**).

Antidepressants

Tricyclic antidepressants
Amongst the TCAs, a recent review found that research has pointed to clomipramine, amitriptyline, and imipramine as the worst offenders, with SD manifesting as decreased desire, lubrication difficulties, and inhibition of ejaculation and orgasm.[74] A double-blind placebo controlled study of 33 subjects with obsessive-compulsive disorder showed that up to 96% of the 24 subjects in the clomipramine group experienced total or partial anorgasmia.[75] Clomipramine has been successfully used to treat premature ejaculation in several studies, including in a 2004 head-to-head randomized, double-blind fixed-dose study of 30 men with lifelong premature ejaculation. Using stop watch assessment, clomipramine was shown to be more effective than paroxetine.[76] Another review found spontaneous orgasms and painful ejaculation with clomipramine.[77] Desipramine and nortriptyline (secondary amines) seem to have lower rates of sexual adverse effects by comparison. A review of case reports also found amoxapine (tetracyclic antidepressant or secondary amine TCA) to be associated with painful and retrograde ejaculation.[74] Overall, some TCAs show high rates of SD, with evidence suggesting that tertiary amines are worse than secondary amines.

Selective Serotonin Reuptake Inhibitors

SD reported with SSRIs includes reduced desire, arousal difficulties (erectile dysfunction, problems with vaginal lubrication), delayed orgasm or anorgasmia, and

Table 1
Evidence for genetic polymorphisms in antidepressant-associated sexual dysfunction

Study, Year	Number of Subjects	Polymorphisms Studied	Subject Population	Agents Studied	Measurement of Sexual Functioning	Major Results	Level of Evidence
Zourkova et al,[56] 2002	30	CYP2D6*1, *3, *4, *5, *6	Men and women with depression	Paroxetine	ASEX	CYP2D6 poor metabolizer phenotype was associated with SD	Level II-2
Zourkova et al,[57] 2007	55	CYP2D6*1, *3, *4, *5, *6	Men and women with anxiety or depression	Paroxetine	ASEX	CYP2D6 poor metabolizer phenotype was associated with SD in women	Level II-2
Bly et al,[58] 2013	57	ABCB1 1236C>T (rs1128503), 2677G>T (rs2032582), 3435C>T (rs1045642) and rs2235015	Women with depression	Citalopram, escitalopram, paroxetine, or sertraline (p-glycoprotein substrates) and fluoxetine (not a p-glycoprotein substrate) as a comparison group	CSFQ	ABCB1 1236 C allele was associated with SD	Level II-2
Zourkova et al,[59] 2013	18	ABCB1 2677G>T (rs2032582) and 3435C>T (rs1045642)	Women with bulimia nervosa	Paroxetine	UKU	ABCB1 2677 G allele was associated with treatment-emergent orgasm and lubrication disorders	Level II-2
Perlis et al,[61] 2003	36	SLC6A4 5HTTLPR	Men and women with MDD	Fluoxetine	Spontaneous subject reports	5HTTLPR genotype was not associated with SD	Level II-2

Study	N	Gene(s)	Population	Medication	Measure	Results	Level
Bishop et al,[60] 2009	101	*SLC6A4* 5HTTLPR and STin2; *HTR2A* −1438A>G (rs6311)	Men and women with depression	Citalopram, escitalopram, fluoxetine, paroxetine, or sertraline	CSFQ	5HTTLPR *L/L* and *HTR2A* −1438 G/G genotypes were associated with SD. STin2 was not associated with SD	Level II-2
Strohmaier et al,[62] 2011	473	*SLC6A4* 5HTTLPR	Men and women with depression	Escitalopram or nortriptyline (TCA)	AAEC, UKU, CSFQ	5HTTLPR was not associated with SD	Level I
Safarinejad,[63] 2010	227	*SLC6A4* 5HTTLPR and STin2	Men with lifelong premature ejaculation	Sertraline	Intravaginal ejaculation latency time	5HTTLPR L_A/L_A and STin2 12/12 were associated with better response	Level II-2
Janssen et al,[64] 2014	54	*SLC6A4* 5HTTLPR	Dutch men with lifelong premature ejaculation	Paroxetine	Intravaginal ejaculation latency time	5HTTLPR was not associated with intravaginal ejaculatory latency time improvement	Level II-2
Bishop et al,[66] 2006	81	*HTR2A* −1438A>G (rs6311), *GNB3* 825C>T (rs5443)	Men and women with depression	Citalopram, escitalopram, fluoxetine, paroxetine, or sertraline	CSFQ	*HTR2A* −1438 G/G genotype was associated with SD. *GNB3* genotype was not associated with SD	Level II-2
Perlis et al,[70] 2009	1473	68 candidate genes related to dopamine, serotonin, adrenergic receptors, glutamate, neurotrophin, as well as other signaling pathways and second-messenger genes	White men and women with MDD	Citalopram	SRIAE	*GRIA3* and *GRIK2* were associated with decreased libido. *GRIA1* was associated with difficulty achieving orgasm. *GRIN3A* was associated with achieving erection	Level II-2

(continued on next page)

Table 1
(continued)

Study, Year	Number of Subjects	Polymorphisms Studied	Subject Population	Agents Studied	Measurement of Sexual Functioning	Major Results	Level of Evidence
Liang et al,[67] 2012	45	HTR2A−1438A>G (rs6311)	Han Chinese men with MDD	SSRI or venlafaxine (SNRI)	ASEX	HTR2A−1438 A/A genotype was associated with SD	Level II-2
Garfield et al,[65] 2014	85	SLC6A4 5HTTLPR, HTR1A−1019C>G (rs6295), HTR2A −1438A>G (rs6311)	Men and women aged >60 y with GAD	Escitalopram	UKU	Diminished sexual desire was associated with the 5HTTLPR L$_A$ allele, HTR1A rs6295 G allele genotype, and HTR2A−1438 A allele	Level I
Masiran et al,[68] 2013	95	HTR2A−1438A>G (rs6311)	Malaysian women with MDD in remission	Fluoxetine, sertraline, fluvoxamine, or escitalopram	MVFSI (desire subscale)	HTR2A genotype was not associated with sexual desire disorder	Level II-2
Zou et al,[69] 2010	295	BDNF Val66Met (rs6265)	Chinese men and women with MDD	Fluoxetine	Subject-reported	Valine-encoding allele associated with decreased sexual desire	Level II-2
Bishop et al,[71] 2012	114	GRIK2 (rs513216 and rs9404130), GRIA3 (rs2269551, rs2285127 and rs550640) and GRIA1 (rs1994862)	Men and women with depression	Citalopram, escitalopram, fluoxetine, paroxetine, or sertraline	CSFQ	Candidate SNPs were not associated with CSFQ total scores GRIA1 rs1994862 was associated with arousal dysfunction	Level II-2

Abbreviations: 5-HTT, serotonin transporter; AAEC, antidepressant adverse-effect checklist; ASEX, Arizona Sexual Experience Scale; CSFQ, Changes in Sexual Functioning Questionnaire; GAD, generalized anxiety disorder; MDD, major depressive disorder; MVFSI, Malay Version of Female Sexual Function Index; PRISE, subject-rated inventory of adverse effects; UKU, Udvalg for Kliniske Undersøgelser adverse effect rating scale.

Adapted from Stevenson JM, Bishop JR. Genetic determinants of selective serotonin reuptake inhibitor related sexual dysfunction. Pharmacogenomics 2014;15(14):1794–5. *Reproduced from* Pharmacogenomics as agreed by Future Medicine Ltd.

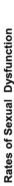
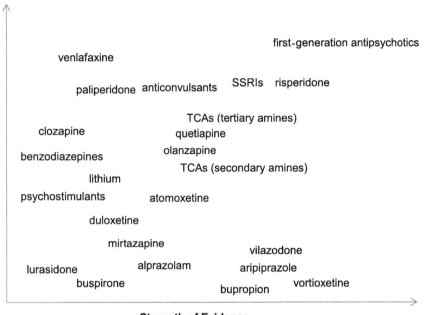

Fig. 2. An approximation of rates of SD with various psychotropics and associated strength of evidence. It would be most appropriate to compare drugs within each class because supporting studies do not compare interclass (ie, TCAs are shown above quetiapine but it may not actually cause higher rates because study populations and comparators are different).

diminished sensation or hyperalgesia. SD associated with fluoxetine was reported just 3 years after its Food and Drug Administration approval. Rates of SD vary widely, approximately 30% to 60% in a 2002 review of 200 studies of all types.[78] Some investigators suggest a higher incidence with certain SSRIs, such as a 2001 prospective multicenter study showing a greater than 70% incidence of SD with citalopram and paroxetine via questionnaire in outpatients with previous normal sexual functioning,[6] whereas another group found no statistically significant differences amongst citalopram, fluoxetine, paroxetine, and sertraline in a cross-sectional observational study of 6297 outpatients receiving antidepressant monotherapy.[79]

Some differences in rates may be related to use of validated questionnaires, rates associated with a single phase of the sexual response cycle versus overall SD, and evaluation of different populations (eg, age, gender). A 2005 retrospective study suggests an improvement in SD after switch from fluoxetine, paroxetine, citalopram, sertraline, and venlafaxine to escitalopram.[80] There have been isolated case reports of increased sexual desire, spontaneous orgasms, and orgasms during exercise with fluoxetine, priapism with citalopram, and increased desire as well as anorgasmia with sertraline.[81] As treatment of premature ejaculation, all SSRIs have been suggested as useful, without any seen as more effective than others. The evidence suggests overall relatively high rates of SD across all the SSRIs.

Serotonin Norepinephrine Reuptake Inhibiters

Most studies looking into serotonin-norepinephrine reuptake inhibitors (SNRIs) have focused on venlafaxine and duloxetine. There have been conflicting reports regarding

SD with venlafaxine. The most reliable figure seems to be in a 2009 meta-analysis that quotes a rate of 80%, among the highest of all the antidepressants examined.[7] There have been some isolated case reports of increased libido, orgasm, and spontaneous erections. Despite the high rate previously mentioned, substantial evidence for venlafaxines use in treatment of premature ejaculation is lacking. In a 2007 double-blind, placebo-controlled comparison trial in subjects with major depressive disorder, no significant differences were found in rates of SD between duloxetine and escitalopram after 12 weeks; however, escitalopram separated from placebo, whereas duloxetine did not.[82] Two comparison studies referred to in a comprehensive review found that duloxetine had lower rates of SD when compared with paroxetine.[81] In summary, it seems that venlafaxine has among the highest rates of SD, whereas duloxetine, in some cases, can be comparable to placebo.

Mirtazapine

Mirtazapine is an antagonist of central presynaptic α_2-adrenergic, 5-HT2, 5-HT3, histamine 1, and muscarinic receptors. Mirtazapine has been reported to cause less SD compared with SSRIs in a large prospective trial, with an incidence of 24.4%, lower than all SSRIs (fluoxetine, 57.7%; sertraline, 62.9%; fluvoxamine, 62.3%; paroxetine, 70.7%) and venlafaxine, 67.3%.[6] An open-label trial in 2000 of 19 subjects in remission from major depressive disorder but experiencing SSRI-induced SD showed evidence for switching from SSRIs to mirtazapine to mitigate SD associated with SSRIs.[83] A randomized, double-blind study in 197 depressed subjects found less SD in the mirtazapine group.[84]

Bupropion

Bupropion is a norepinephrine-dopamine reuptake inhibitor. It seems to have one of the lowest rates of SD, with rates ranging from 3% to 14% in a review of 10 studies,[81] and 10% in a 2009 meta-analysis.[7] Bupropion has been shown to improve sexual adverse effects in 2 studies: a 1985 prospective study that showed improvement in 24 of 48 men experiencing SD on previous antidepressants[85] and a 2006 prospective open-label study of 18 women experiencing SD with SSRIs.[86] Overall, there is considerable evidence to suggest SD at or below the rate of placebo exists for bupropion.[81]

Other Antidepressants

An examination of short-term studies (3829 subjects) showed that SD with vortioxetine was not statistically higher when compared with placebo, and was statistically lower compared with duloxetine (37% vs 42%).[87] In a randomized, double-blind trial of 447 subjects with major depression experiencing SD with SSRIs or SNRIs (most commonly citalopram), cross-titration to vortioxetine or escitalopram showed improvement in both groups but statistically greater improvement in SD with vortioxetine, as evaluated by the CSFQ, in all 3 phases of sexual function.[88]

Phenelzine, isocarboxazid, and tranylcypromine are all irreversible monoamine oxidase inhibitors. Limited evidence exists about SD with their use but 3 papers in a 2014 review suggest an incidence of SD of 20% to 40%,[81] whereas another estimates a higher rate at 42%.[7] There has been 1 documented case of priapism with phenelzine.[89] In a 2008 review, transdermal selegiline was shown to have rates of SD comparable to placebo.[90]

Trazodone, a serotonin transporter inhibitor and 5-HT2A/2C receptor antagonist, has shown increased sexual desire according to 2 sets of case reports, 3 men and 3 women total, written in the 1980s.[81,91,92] There have been several reports of priapism in individual case studies; however, overall reports of SD seem to be low.[81]

In a year-long, open-label study using the CSFQ to determine the rate of SD in 869 subjects with major depression treated with vilazodone, a serotonin transport modulator and 5-HT1A receptor partial agonist, no significant difference from placebo was seen.[93]

Anticonvulsant Mood Stabilizers

Much of the data surrounding SD with mood stabilizers are derived from the neurology literature. Overall, the incidence of SD with the use of mood stabilizers has not been well studied in subjects with primary psychiatric disorders. Again, it is important to note that there is a wide range of sexual problems in patients with epilepsy, which may confound the assessment of SD with anticonvulsants and mood stabilizers. Overall, the older agents, for example, carbamazepine, phenytoin, have all been associated with SD, with the idea that patients taking the anticonvulsants had lower bioavailable testosterone secondary to induced hepatic metabolism of sex hormone binding globulin.[42] Carbamazepine, in a cross-sectional study of men with epilepsy, was associated with significant erectile dysfunction compared with healthy controls and was also associated with lower testosterone levels.[94] In 4 case studies, decreased libido, and anorgasmia were reported by women with bipolar disorder taking divalproex, a drug that has otherwise been viewed as free of SD.[40] Another isolated case report describes retrograde ejaculation in a patient on divalproex who was also taking phenytoin.[95] There is conflicting evidence with oxcarbazepine in patients with epilepsy[52] and, unfortunately, no studies have been published looking at SD in subjects taking oxcarbazepine off-label to treat mood disorders. SD with lamotrigine was equivalent to normal controls and superior to carbamazepine and phenytoin after 6 months of treatment in a nonrandomized, observational, cross-sectional study of 85 men with localization-related epilepsy.[53] Overall, it seems that anticonvulsants that do not cause hepatic enzyme induction produce less SD than those that do. Lamotrigine seems to be the anticonvulsant least associated with SD in the epilepsy literature.

Lithium

Lithium, primarily used for the treatment of psychiatric disorders, has been poorly studied with regard to SD.[36] A 1987 retrospective study found 6 of 24 subjects treated with lithium had changes in sexual function, 5 negative and 1 positive.[96] In a 1992 observational study in subjects with bipolar disorder, SD was significantly higher in subjects cotreated with benzodiazepines (49%), compared with the lithium monotherapy group (14%) and lithium in combination with other psychotropics (17%).[97] An open-label study in 1992 reported 31% SD in 35 subjects treated with lithium for bipolar or schizoaffective disorders.[37]

Anxiolytics

A 2014 review cites 8 studies, primarily case reports and retrospective studies, describing decreased sexual desire and delayed orgasm with the use of the benzodiazepines diazepam, clonazepam, lorazepam, and alprazolam.[52] A double-blind randomized trial in 190 subjects with panic disorder aiming to assess sexual function showed no significant difference before and after treatment with alprazolam.[98] Buspirone, a 5-HT1A partial agonist has been shown to reverse sexual adverse effects of SSRIs at higher doses but studies have yet to be replicated.[52]

Antipsychotics

Antipsychotic medications can contribute to SD in all 3 phases of sexual response,[74] despite the high prevalence of SD at baseline that occurs with disorders like schizophrenia.[99] First-generation antipsychotics, specifically chlorpromazine, pimozide, thioridazine, and thiothixene have been associated with decreased sexual desire and erectile dysfunction.[100] Multiple case reports reviewed point toward thioridazine, with the highest frequency of SD, followed by trifluoperazine. Priapism occurs with all antipsychotics,[101] with cases specifically reported with aripiprazole, clozapine, olanzapine, quetiapine, risperidone, and ziprasidone.[99]

A 2009 meta-analysis described a lower rate of SD with the prolactin-sparing antipsychotics quetiapine, ziprasidone, perphenazine, and aripiprazole (16%–27%) compared with prolactin-raising antipsychotics olanzapine, risperidone, haloperidol, clozapine, and thioridazine (40%–60%).[102] Although olanzapine is often included as a prolactogenic drug, it seems that prolactin elevations were transient, returning to baseline levels after 6 weeks of treatment with the highest elevations below levels seen with haloperidol.[99,103] This may explain its location below risperidone and the conventional antipsychotic medications with respect to SD. A study assessing 199 subjects with psychotic illness found that risperidone and first-generation agents had higher rates of decreased libido and dysorgasmia compared with antipsychotics that are not prolactogenic.[104] A randomized, double-blind comparison study of 27 subjects with schizophrenia showed high rates of SD with fluphenazine (78%), quetiapine (50%), and risperidone (42%) in subjects with schizophrenia; however, only quetiapine showed improvement in the arousal phase.[105] An open-label comparison study in 46 subjects showed lower frequency of SD with olanzapine (12%) versus risperidone (52%).[104] A prospective study also found 46% of 243 subjects with psychotic illnesses reporting SD, with typical antipsychotics and risperidone having a significantly increased risk of SD compared with olanzapine.[106] An observational study of 636 subjects with schizophrenia further corroborated this, with less SD in subjects taking quetiapine (18%) versus olanzapine (35%), haloperidol (38%), and risperidone (43%).[107]

Despite these positive studies linking antipsychotics that elevate prolactin levels with SD, several negative studies[74,108,109] and 1 observational study with 3838 subjects have shown no statistically significant differences between haloperidol (71%), risperidone (68%), quetiapine (60%), olanzapine (56%).[110] A cross-sectional observational study in 827 clinically stable subjects with schizophrenia treated with greater than 1 antipsychotic medication experienced more SD than those taking any single second-generation antipsychotic. In this study, women on antipsychotics experienced the same level (68%) of SD as healthy controls.[111]

Aripiprazole seems to have the lowest incidence of SD compared with other antipsychotics in subjects with schizophrenia.[112] There was also reported improvement in delayed ejaculation and orgasm in a 42-subject observational study.[113] As an augmentation agent to antidepressants such as SSRIs, SNRIs, and bupropion, aripiprazole resulted in improvement in depression and SD assessed with the Massachusetts General Hospital Sexual Functioning Inventory at 52 weeks.[114] Several other comparison studies included in a 2014 review of risperidone, olanzapine, and haloperidol report less SD in aripiprazole as a tertiary outcome.[74] Overall, in these comparison studies, it seems that SD occurs with all antipsychotics, with the highest rates in prolactogenic drugs, first-generation antipsychotics along with risperidone, followed by olanzapine and clozapine, then quetiapine, and finally, aripiprazole.[74]

Paliperidone, the active metabolite of risperidone, was shown to have prolactin elevations similar to its parent compound, risperidone.[115] However, a small prospective observational study in 11 subjects showed a 4-fold reduction in significant SD after switching from long-acting injectable risperidone to injectable paliperidone palmitate.[116] Similarly, a case report showed decreased SD in a patient with schizophrenia who switched from oral risperidone to paliperidone.[117]

Clozapine has been noted to have high rates of SD but lower rates than olanzapine, risperidone, quetiapine, and typical antipsychotic medications.[118] A 1999 prospective study in 153 subjects with schizophrenia found no significant difference in rates of SD between clozapine and haloperidol.[99] There have been several case reports of priapism.[119] A small study of 9 subjects with schizophrenia found that the primary sexual complaint was decreased ejaculatory volume.[120] Clozapine has not been associated with prolactin elevations.[99] Finally, a study looking at pretreatment and post-treatment SD in depressed subjects with lurasidone found significantly greater (14%) reduction of sexual symptoms versus 9% with placebo.[114] No studies have been published regarding iloperidone-induced SD outside of 1 case report of retrograde ejaculation.[121]

Psychostimulants and Atomoxetine

Very little is known about SD in treatments for attention deficit hyperactivity disorder (ADHD). A pooled analysis of 3314 subjects with ADHD treated with atomoxetine found that adult men reported more sexual and genitourinary adverse effects with atomoxetine when compared with placebo, including libido decrease (4.6% vs 3%, respectively), ejaculation disorder (2.8% vs 1.1%, respectively), and erectile dysfunction as the most common (8.0% vs 1.9%, respectively).[122] Very little information exists for SD associated with methylphenidate outside of a case report of a 14-year-old who experienced priapism[122] and another who had spontaneous ejaculation.[123] There have been reports of spontaneous erections and hypersexuality with osmotic-release oral system methylphenidate.[124] Although much has been written about the contribution of acute use of illicit stimulants to sexual desire, little has been written about SD in the setting of controlled, chronic amphetamine use in treating ADHD.

TREATMENT OF MEDICATION-ASSOCIATED SEXUAL DYSFUNCTION

Given the prevalence of medication-induced SD, finding effective management of this adverse effect is of paramount importance due to the concern for medication noncompliance. Fortunately, there are many different treatment strategies available, including both pharmacologic and nonpharmacologic options (**Fig. 3**). Although only a small percentage of the studies that have been done thus far on medication-induced SD have resulted in data with strong statistical significance,[125] all of the options proposed here warrant clinical consideration for patients on a case-by-case basis.

Many clinicians opt to start with a medication known to have a lower incidence of sexual adverse effects in patients experiencing sexual difficulties related to their psychiatric condition or who have concerns about developing SD. When a patient is experiencing medication-induced SD, the 2 most commonly used treatment strategies are switching to a medication that is known to have a lower incidence of sexual adverse effects or adding a medication that can help to reverse the SD. Other pharmacologic strategies include waiting for spontaneous resolution of the adverse effects, lowering the medication dose, or having the patient take intermittent drug holidays. Nonpharmacologic options include psychotherapy (individual and/or couples), modification of sexual technique, scheduling regular sexual activity, and exercise before sexual activity.

Waiting for Spontaneous Remission

Many clinicians choose to wait for possible remission of sexual adverse effects before making any changes to the patient's regimen. There are case reports about

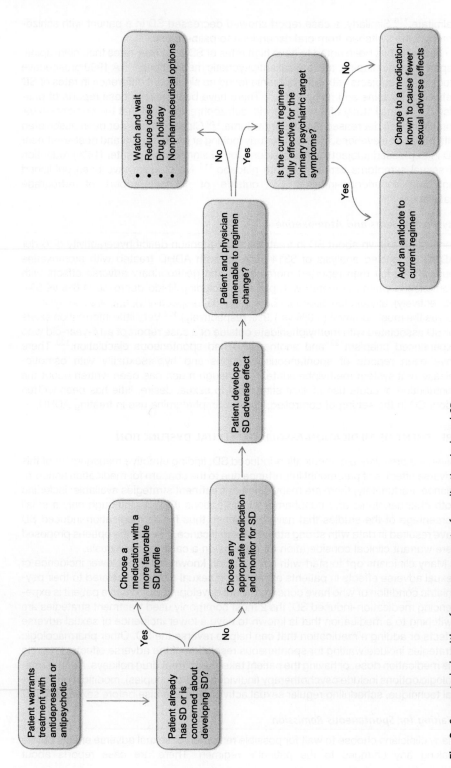

Fig. 3. Suggested algorithm for management of medication-induced SD.

spontaneous remission of antidepressant-induced SD,[126,127] although studies have largely found that spontaneous remission not only takes 4 to 6 months to occur but also occurs in only 5% to 10% of subjects.[6,128,129] Waiting for spontaneous remission of sexual adverse effects may result in an increased likelihood of medication noncompliance or a disruption in the patient-physician relationship and ongoing treatment.

Dose Reduction

SD caused by SSRIs is both dose-dependent and reversible.[8] Therefore, reducing the dose of the medication can be an effective strategy, although careful clinical monitoring for potential relapse of psychiatric symptoms would be prudent if taking this approach.

Drug Holiday

A drug holiday, in which the patient does not take the medication for 2 to 3 days before sexual activity, can be an effective strategy for those participating in infrequent and planned sexual activity but carries the risk of SSRI discontinuation syndrome symptoms and increases the risk of the patient stopping the medication entirely, which could result in relapse of mood symptoms.[130] Only 1 open label study has been conducted and it found that when subjects skipped 2 consecutive doses of either sertraline or paroxetine each weekend for 4 consecutive weekends, there was an improvement in sexual functioning on the days that the medication was not taken. This strategy was not effective for subjects taking fluoxetine, likely because of its longer half-life. The study did not find evidence of worsening of depressive symptoms during this 4-week period. It did not evaluate emergence of SSRI discontinuation syndrome symptoms. Unfortunately, this strategy is unlikely to be a satisfactory permanent solution for many patients because SD has a very high likelihood of reoccurrence when the medication is restarted.[131]

Nonpharmacologic Interventions

There have been no randomized trials evaluating the effectiveness of nonpharmacologic treatments for medication-induced SD[125] but these strategies may be a good first step if the clinician or patient is hesitant to make a change to the existing medication regimen. If there are any psychological factors contributing to the SD (eg, performance anxiety, interpersonal conflict with sexual partner, history of sexual trauma) the patient may benefit from psychotherapy (individual and/or couples). Exercise before sexual activity may result in an increase in sexual desire[132] and engaging in regularly scheduled sexual activity may improve orgasm function in women.[133] Additionally, changing sexual technique (eg, position, activity) can sometimes be helpful. Although these strategies may not be as effective as pharmacologic intervention, they may be helpful in an augmenting role if used in conjunction with a change to the medication regimen.

Switching to a Different Antidepressant

Antidepressants that seem to be associated with a lower incidence of sexual adverse effects include bupropion, mirtazapine, vilazodone, vortioxetine, nefazodone, agomelatine, and moclobemide.[7,79,81,134–137] Although older comparative studies did not find any statistically significant difference in the rate of SD among the SSRIs,[79,131,138–141] a recent meta-analysis was able to quantify the risk of SD with certain medications, with the stratification being as follows (from least likely to most likely to cause SD): moclobemide (4%), agomelatine (4%), amineptine (7%), nefazodone (8%), bupropion (10%), mirtazapine (24%), fluvoxamine (26%), escitalopram (37%), duloxetine (42%), phenelzine (42%), imipramine (44%), fluoxetine (70%), paroxetine (71%), citalopram (79%), venlafaxine (80%).[7] Switching to a different medication may lead to a less effective treatment response, so depressive symptoms and sexual function should be monitored (**Table 2**).

Bupropion

Numerous studies have demonstrated that bupropion has a markedly more favorable sexual adverse effect profile than other antidepressants.[7,142–153] Both the extended release (XL) and sustained release (SR) formulations have demonstrated superiority compared with SSRIs in terms of sexual adverse effect profile. Bupropion XL (300–450 mg/day) was found to cause significantly less sexual adverse effects than escitalopram (10–20 mg/day) and did not cause more sexual adverse effects than placebo.[146] Bupropion SR (150–400 mg/day) was found to cause significantly less sexual adverse effects than sertraline (50–200 mg/day)[149,150] or fluoxetine (20–60 mg/day).[147] Additionally, although several SSRIs have been found to negatively interfere with orgasm and ejaculation, bupropion was not associated with that adverse effect.[128,147] Notably, in the 2013 Cochrane review on treatment strategies for antidepressant-induced SD, bupropion was the only medication, aside from as-needed sildenafil, found to have strong data with statistical significance for reversing treatment-emergent SD in both men and women.[125]

Mirtazapine

Mirtazapine has been associated with lower rates of sexual adverse effects than SSRIs,[6,83,84,153,154] and it may help to alleviate medication-induced SD if added to

---

Table 2
Medications with favorable SD profiles and SD antidotes

More Favorable SD Profile	Antidote
Treatment of antidepressant-induced SD	
Bupropion[a]	Bupropion[a]
Vortioxetine[a]	PDE-5 inhibitor[a]
Mirtazapine	Mirtazapine
Vilazodone	—
Desvenlafaxine	—
Agomelatine	—
Moclobemide	—
Nefazodone	—
Treatment of antipsychotic-induced SD	
Aripiprazole[a]	Aripiprazole[a]
Quetiapine	PDE-5 inhibitor (men only)[a]
Ziprasidone	—
Clozapine	—
Olanzapine	—

Medications that have level 1 evidence to support that they either have a more favorable SD profile (known to cause less sexual adverse effects) or are effective at treating the sexual adverse effects caused by other medications when used in an adjunctive role. In making treatment choices, managing the primary psychiatric symptoms should always take priority.
Abbreviation: PDE-5, phosphodiesterase type 5.
[a] Medications with level 1A (highest level) evidence.

the current medication regimen.[155,156] One uncontrolled study found that switching from an SSRI to mirtazapine resulted in a decrease in antidepressant-induced SD.[83]

Vilazodone
Vilazodone is an SSRI and 5-HT 1A partial agonist that has only been compared with 1 other antidepressant in a head-to-head trial evaluating sexual adverse effects.[157] In this study, women taking vilazodone or placebo had more improvement in CSFQ scores than women taking citalopram; but no inferential statistics were performed.[157] However, in the placebo-controlled studies with vilazodone, it seems that vilazodone has a rate of sexual adverse effects comparable to placebo.[93,137,158–160]

Vortioxetine
Vortioxetine is a newer antidepressant that is a serotonin reuptake inhibitor and a 5-HT receptor modulator (agonist at 5-HT1A, partial agonist at 5-HT1B, and antagonist of 5-HT3, 5-HT1D, and 5-HT7 receptors). It has been suggested that vortioxetine may have a lower incidence of sexual adverse effects.[161] A pooled analysis of 7 studies demonstrated that vortioxetine has been found equivalent to placebo in the risk of causing either new symptoms of SD or worsening of pre-existing symptoms of SD.[87] Another study found that subjects with SSRI-induced SD on citalopram, paroxetine, or sertraline had significantly greater improvement in sexual functioning when their medication was switched to vortioxetine versus switching to escitalopram.[88] However, in more than half of these subjects, the antidepressant that was associated with the SD was citalopram, which may have biased the study in favor of vortioxetine.

Desvenlafaxine
In a randomized, double-blind, placebo-controlled study, both male and female subjects received either placebo or the SNRI desvenlafaxine 50 mg/day and, after 12 weeks of treatment, the rate of SD was statistically equivalent between desvenlafaxine and placebo. The only exception was new onset orgasmic dysfunction at week 12 in men who did not have SD before starting desvenlafaxine.[162] A recent post hoc analysis of pooled data from 3 randomized, double-blind, placebo-controlled studies evaluating the rate of SD in subjects treated with desvenlafaxine 50 mg/day or 100 mg/day found that desvenlafaxine did not have a statistically significant effect on sexual function versus placebo, although there was a greater incidence of reported sexual adverse effects at 100 mg compared with 50 mg.[163]

Nefazodone
Nefazodone is a serotonin reuptake inhibitor and a 5-HT2 antagonist. Several studies have found that nefazodone is associated with a low rate of SD.[6,164–166] More specifically, in 1 study nefazodone was found to have a low incidence of sexual adverse effects overall and had notably less sexual adverse effects than citalopram, paroxetine, sertraline, fluvoxamine, fluoxetine, or venlafaxine.[6] Another study found that switching from sertraline to nefazodone resulted in a reduced occurrence of antidepressant-induced SD.[131] Of note, the use of nefazodone in the United States, both clinically and in studies, has been very low over the past decade due to the warning regarding hepatotoxicity.

Agomelatine
Agomelatine is an agonist at melatonin MT1 and MT2 receptors and a 5-HT2C antagonist. Studies have found that the rate of SD is low with agomelatine and that it specifically has a more favorable sexual adverse effect profile than venlafaxine[143] and escitalopram.[135]

Moclobemide

Moclobemide, a reversible monoamine oxidase-A inhibitor, has consistently been found to have a favorable profile in terms of sexual adverse effects.[139,167–170] Specific studies have found that moclobemide has lower rates of SD than venlafaxine, paroxetine, and sertraline[167] and that moclobemide results in increased sexual desire as compared with doxepin.[171]

Reboxetine

Reboxetine, a norepinephrine reuptake inhibitor, seems to have a lower likelihood of causing SD, although the published data are not definitive.[172–175] Nonetheless, reboxetine seems to have less sexual adverse effects than fluoxetine, citalopram, and paroxetine,[172–174] and seems to be associated with greater sexual satisfaction than fluoxetine.[172]

Trazodone

Trazodone carries a low risk for inducing SD and may in fact have positive effects on sexual functioning by increasing desire.[91,92] A recent comparative study found that trazodone was associated with fewer sexual adverse effects than fluoxetine and sertraline.[176]

Tianeptine

Tianeptine is an antidepressant similar to the TCAs that is also a μ-opioid and σ-opioid agonist, and adenosine A1 receptor agonist. In an open label study, subjects experiencing sexual adverse effects from clomipramine, paroxetine, sertraline, or fluoxetine experienced resolution of those adverse effects when they switched to tianeptine.[177]

Selegiline

The transdermal formulation of selegiline, a newer irreversible monoamine oxidase inhibitor, has a low incidence of SD versus placebo.[90]

Adding a Medication to Treat Sexual Adverse Effects

If the current medication regimen is working well (aside from the sexual adverse effects), both the clinician and patient may be appropriately hesitant to change to a different medication. In that instance, adding another medication to the current regimen to counteract sexual adverse effects may be a good strategy to consider. Based on the available evidence, the only treatment strategies with clear statistically significant benefit include switching to or adding bupropion in men or women, or adding a phosphodiesterase inhibitor in men.[125] Many other medications have been studied in an augmentation role for treatment of antidepressant-induced SD, including mirtazapine, buspirone, antihistamines, amantadine, yohimbine, aripiprazole, bethanechol, granisetron, and adenosylmethionine, as well as several herbal medications, including ginkgo biloba, Rosa damascena oil, and maca root.[178–180] Some of these, however, have little or no evidence of their effectiveness.

Bupropion

Adding bupropion, a norepinephrine-dopamine reuptake inhibitor, to the current medication regimen may help to alleviate antidepressant-induced sexual adverse effects and may also have the added benefit of enhancing treatment of depressive symptoms. Addition of bupropion to an established regimen may help to reverse medication-induced SD by increasing sexual desire and improving overall sexual functioning.[181–184] Although some randomized controlled trials were negative, the Cochrane review from 2013 concluded that bupropion was efficacious as an antidote for antidepressant-associated SD.[125] The effectiveness is clearly dose-related in that daily doses of 150 mg were often not sufficient but at doses of 300 to 450 mg per day there was benefit in improvement in SD.[183,185–188]

Phosphodiesterase type 5 inhibitors: sildenafil and tadalafil
The use of sildenafil before sexual activity is effective at reversing antidepressant-induced arousal and orgasmic dysfunction in men[189,190] and women.[191] In the 2013 Cochrane review, sildenafil was the only medication, aside from bupropion, that was considered to have strong supportive evidence for its use as an adjunctive treatment of medication-induced SD.[125]

One prospective, double-blind, randomized study demonstrated improvement in erectile function in men when tadalafil 10 to 20 mg was taken just before sexual activity.[192]

Mirtazapine
Some data have investigated whether adding mirtazapine to an SSRI reduces SSRI-induced SD.[155,193,194] However, this has yet to be shown in a randomized, controlled clinical trial. A potential benefit from adding mirtazapine to an SSRI may be further improvement in depressive symptoms.[155,156]

Buspirone
There have not been many studies done on the use of adjunctive buspirone, a 5-HT1A partial agonist, although it is commonly used in clinical practice as an additive agent for treatment of SSRI-induced SD. One study found buspirone to be effective when added to either citalopram or paroxetine for the reversal of SSRI-induced SD.[195] Another study did not find it to be efficacious when added to fluoxetine.[196] This combination may also improve depressive symptoms.[197]

Antihistaminic agents: cyproheptadine and loratadine
A recent case report cited reversal of SSRI-induced anorgasmia in 4 women who took cyproheptadine as needed 30 to 60 minutes before sexual activity.[198] Before that, there had been several case reports of men finding improvement in SSRI-induced SD with administration of as-needed cyproheptadine.[199–201] The main concern with cyproheptadine is its potential for interfering with the antidepressant properties of SSRIs if taken on a daily basis, due to its antiserotonergic properties.[202]

One open-label study administered loratadine 10 mg/day to 9 male subjects experiencing SSRI-induced erectile dysfunction and found statistically significant improvement in erectile function after 2 weeks.[203]

Amantadine
Amantadine is an antiviral agent that is also a dopamine agonist, N-methyl-d-aspartate receptor antagonist, and is antimuscarinic. Several older studies found that adding amantadine reduces SD caused by SSRIs,[178,204–206] although other adverse effects may occur. In the most recent study done on augmentation with amantadine, adding 50 mg twice daily was not found to be effective.[178]

Yohimbine
Yohimbine is a presynaptic α2-adrenergic antagonist and agonist at 5-HT1a, 5-HT1B, 5-HT 1D, and D2 receptors. It seems to be more effective than amantadine at reversing medication-induced SD.[207] Two studies evaluated augmentation with yohimbine, and although many patients reported improvement in SD, the results were not statistically significant.[125,193]

Bethanecol

One study found that taking bethanecol 20 mg 45 minutes before sexual activity was effective for clomipramine-induced orgasmic dysfunction in 12 male subjects.[208] Bethanecol has primarily been studied as an adjunct to TCAs, because the cholinergic properties of bethanecol seem to help reverse the anticholinergic properties of TCAs that result in SD.[209,210]

Granisetron

Adding granisetron (a 5-HT3 agonist) was evaluated in 2 studies and, although it may be helpful, the data were not definitive and suggested a possible placebo response in subjects who found benefit.[211,212]

Adenosylmethionine

One study found that the addition of s-adenosylmethionine improved medication-induced erectile dysfunction in men.[213]

Herbals

Adding ginkgo biloba was evaluated in 2 studies of SSRI-induced SD but was not found to be more effective than placebo.[214,215] Adding Rosa damascena oil may help to reverse SSRI-induced SD, mainly in men.[216,217] Maca root may help to alleviate SSRI-induced SD[218] and may be specifically beneficial in postmenopausal women.[219]

ANTIPSYCHOTICS

Not as commonly recognized but arguably equally prevalent are sexual adverse effects caused by antipsychotic medications. The body of research on treatment of antipsychotic-induced SD is notably small and frequently inconsistent. Nonetheless, treatment of sexual adverse effects in patients with schizophrenia or other psychotic illnesses is extremely important because SD may contribute to difficulties with social functioning and nonadherence to treatment. Therefore, SD should be regularly assessed in patients on antipsychotics and if sexual adverse effects do occur clinical management is advised (see **Table 2**).

The treatment strategies for antipsychotic-induced SD are similar to the strategies for antidepressant-induced SD. Waiting for spontaneous remission or tolerance to antipsychotic-induced sexual adverse effects has not been formally studied but this is a potential first-step option. Dose reduction requires close monitoring for relapse of psychotic symptoms, and drug holidays are not recommended due to concerns for medication discontinuation. The recommended strategies are starting with or switching to an antipsychotic that carries a lower incidence of SD or adding a medication to the regimen that may reverse the sexual adverse effects.

Lower Incidence of Sexual Dysfunction

If an increase in prolactin was the only mechanism of action by which antipsychotics caused SD, it could be assumed that a lower incidence of SD would be associated with the prolactin-sparing antipsychotics (aripiprazole, clozapine, olanzapine, quetiapine, ziprasidone).[74] However, to date, the research done on this topic has resulted in data that are highly variable. In a recent meta-analysis, lower rates of sexual adverse effects were found in aripiprazole, quetiapine, ziprasidone, and perphenazine, whereas higher rates were seen in clozapine, olanzapine risperidone, haloperidol, and thioridazine.[102] A literature review conducted in 2003 found that clozapine, olanzapine, quetiapine, and sertindole had lower rates of SD than risperidone and typical antipsychotics.[72] In contrast, an observational study of 3838 subjects found that there was no statistically significant difference in the prevalence of sexual adverse effects between olanzapine, quetiapine, risperidone, and haldoperidol.[110]

Although the aforementioned studies suggest quetiapine may have a lower propensity for sexual adverse effects, there are some inconsistencies in the data. A cross-sectional study found that quetiapine was associated with a lower rate of SD than olanzapine, haloperidol, and risperidone[107]; however, several other studies have contradicted this finding. One study found that switching from risperidone to quetiapine did not result in improvement in sexual adverse effects, although the sample size was notably small (22 subjects).[108] Other studies found there was no statistical significance in the difference between the sexual adverse effects of quetiapine compared with olanzapine and risperidone.[109,110,220,221]

There is some evidence that olanzapine may be superior to risperidone and typical antipsychotics in terms of sexual adverse effect profile. One study found that switching to olanzapine from risperidone resulted in improvement in sexual desire.[222] Another study found that olanzapine caused less SD than risperidone.[104] In a 4-month, open-label, prospective study, both male and female subjects with stable schizophrenia treated with either risperidone or a typical antipsychotic were either maintained on their current regimen or switched to olanzapine. At the end of the study period, subjects who switched to olanzapine had a significant reduction in prolactin levels. Male subjects had an increase in free testosterone, and some female subjects experienced re-regulation of their menstrual cycles and resolution of galactorrhea and gynecomastia. Both genders experienced statistically significant improvement in sexual functioning.[223]

Aripiprazole is the only antipsychotic that has strong evidence to support its favorable profile in terms of sexual adverse effects.[224] Not only does aripiprazole carry a lower risk of SD, it also may, to some degree, reverse the sexual adverse effects caused by both antipsychotics and antidepressants. An open-label study evaluated the impact that either switching to aripiprazole or adding aripiprazole to a pre-established antipsychotic regimen would have on sexual functioning in both men and women. The results at week 12 showed significant reduction in prolactin levels for both groups, with concordant improvement in erectile and ejaculatory function in men and re-regulation of the menstrual cycle in women. With these improvements came an overall improvement in sexual functioning and satisfaction that remained significant when reassessed at week 26.[225] Another open-label study found that depressive symptoms and sexual functioning improved with adjunctive aripiprazole in subjects taking bupropion, an SSRI, or an SNRI for major depressive disorder.[114]

Adding a Medication to Reverse Sexual Dysfunction

As previously noted, aripiprazole has been found to effectively treat sexual adverse effects caused by antipsychotics, likely by reversing hyperprolactinemia.[225]

In a randomized, double-blind, placebo-controlled trial evaluating the addition of as-needed sildenafil for men experiencing antipsychotic-induced erectile dysfunction, there was statistically significant improvement in adequate erections and sexual satisfaction in the sildenafil group over placebo.[226]

In the same way that cholinergic drugs, such as bethanecol and neostigmine, improve anticholinergic-based SD caused by TCAs,[208–210] they can also possibly improve SD caused by the anticholinergic properties of antipsychotics. Similarly, SD caused by the antidopaminergic effects of antipsychotics should theoretically improve with the addition of a dopaminergic medication, such as amantadine, bromocriptine, or cabergoline. However, adding a dopaminergic medication could worsen psychosis, so this option should not be a first-line choice.

SUMMARY

SD is a multifaceted phenomenon. With the current prevalence of mental illness and the difficulty in deciphering if SD is due to the illness itself or to medication, constant vigilance by the prescriber and a keen investigative eye is required. Currently, a great deal remains to be understood about SD from a neurochemical and neuroanatomical perspective. Knowledge of neuroimaging has allowed a glimpse into the neural pathways implicated in sexual function and dysfunction. This is not to minimize the effects psychology has on healthy sexual functioning. Similar to other aspects of mental health, form (biological) and function (psychological) play equally important roles in this area of focus. Based on current knowledge of the neurochemical aspects of sexual functioning, clinicians are now much better equipped to delineate how psychotropic medications affect sexual functioning. Dopamine plays a vital role in healthy sexual functioning with serotonin and norepinephrine playing similarly pivotal roles. With this understanding, it is not difficult to hypothesize how several of the most commonly prescribed psychotropic medications have sexual adverse effects. The prescriber must look beyond interactions with neurotransmitters and also look to the complexity of liver metabolism and pharmacodynamics. For instance, several mood stabilizers affect the liver's production of proteins used to bind hormones, such as testosterone for transportation. Despite having a certain level of understanding, there is still a great deal left unclear about how certain medications (eg, lithium) and classes of medications (eg, benzodiazepines) affect sexual functioning. Research moves onward looking to fMRI and genetic studies of SNPs to gain a better understanding of how psychotropic medications affect sexual functioning.

Overall, evidence for the incidence of medication-associated SD is limited, at best, because most studies measure SD as a tertiary outcome and often without validated scales. Given differing cultural norms and willingness to report SD, it is often understudied and likely underreported. These factors weaken the existing evidence about drug-associated SD.

Based on the available evidence, it seems that bupropion and mirtazapine have the lowest reported rates of SD. SSRIs and TCAs, as classes, seem to have a high incidence of SD. Newer agents with differences in mechanism of action, such as vilazodone and vortioxetine, show promise, with some evidence suggesting low rates of SD. Among the mood stabilizers, anticonvulsants, especially those that lower bioavailable testosterone, seem to have a stronger link to SD, with very little written about lithium. Evidence for benzodiazepines is limited. With antipsychotics, there is good evidence for drug-associated SD in prolactogenic medications, such as first-generation antipsychotics, risperidone, and paliperidone. Lower rates of SD are seen with aripiprazole and lurasidone. Little evidence is available on prescription psychostimulants.

Clinicians are encouraged to always be thinking about and monitoring for SD because it can contribute to worsening depression, anxiety, interpersonal relationships, and social functioning. If a patient is experiencing SD as part of their psychiatric illness or if they are highly worried about the possible impact that developing SD may have on them, choosing a medication known to have a lower likelihood of causing SD is a reasonable first step. Treating the presenting psychiatric symptoms should always take priority and, if the most appropriate medication to treat those symptoms has a high likelihood of causing SD, other management strategies can be used. There is strong evidence for adding a medication that is known to diminish or reverse the sexual adverse effects caused by antidepressants and antipsychotics to the offending regimen. Many other strategies exist, including waiting for spontaneous remission of the sexual adverse effects, lowering the medication dose, implementing intermittent drug holidays, and several nonpharmacologic options, including psychotherapy, modification of sexual technique, scheduling regular sexual activity, and exercise before sexual activity. Even though there is not yet strong evidence behind every treatment option available, the body of research continues to expand and the strategies discussed in this article are all worth considering on a clinical case-by-case basis.

REFERENCES

1. Statistics NCFH. Health, United States, 2012: with special feature on emergency care. Hyattsville (MD): 2013. Available at: www.cdc.gov/nchs/data/hus/hus12. pdf. Accessed May 26, 2016.
2. Abbing-Karahagopian V, Huerta C, Souverein PC, et al. Antidepressant prescribing in five European countries: application of common definitions to assess the prevalence, clinical observations, and methodological implications. Eur J Clin Pharmacol 2014;70(7):849–57.
3. Vilhelmsson A. Depression and antidepressants: a Nordic perspective. Front Public Health 2013;1:30.
4. Arroll B, Macgillivray S, Ogston S, et al. Efficacy and tolerability of tricyclic antidepressants and SSRIs compared with placebo for treatment of depression in primary care: a meta-analysis. Ann Fam Med 2005;3(5):449–56.
5. Bull SA, Hu XH, Hunkeler EM, et al. Discontinuation of use and switching of antidepressants: influence of patient-physician communication. JAMA 2002; 288(11):1403–9.
6. Montejo AL, Llorca G, Izquierdo JA, et al. Incidence of sexual dysfunction associated with antidepressant agents: a prospective multicenter study of 1022 outpatients. Spanish Working Group for the Study of Psychotropic-Related Sexual Dysfunction. J Clin Psychiatry 2001;62(Suppl 3):10–21.
7. Serretti A, Chiesa A. Treatment-emergent sexual dysfunction related to antidepressants: a meta-analysis. J Clin Psychopharmacol 2009;29(3):259–66.
8. Waldinger MD. Psychiatric disorders and sexual dysfunction. Handb Clin Neurol 2015;130:469–89.
9. Zemishlany Z, Weizman A. The impact of mental illness on sexual dysfunction. Adv Psychosom Med 2008;29:89–106.
10. Ishak WW, Christensen S, Sayer G, et al. Sexual satisfaction and quality of life in major depressive disorder before and after treatment with citalopram in the STAR*D study. J Clin Psychiatry 2013;74(3):256–61.
11. Thakurta RG, Singh OP, Bhattacharya A, et al. Nature of sexual dysfunctions in major depressive disorder and its impact on quality of life. Indian J Psychol Med 2012;34(4):365–70.
12. Clayton AH, Croft HA, Handiwala L. Antidepressants and sexual dysfunction: mechanisms and clinical implications. Postgrad Med 2014;126(2):91–9.
13. Graf H, Walter M, Metzger CD, et al. Antidepressant-related sexual dysfunction - perspectives from neuroimaging. Pharmacol Biochem Behav 2014;121:138–45.
14. Stahl SM. The psychopharmacology of sex, part 2: effects of drugs and disease on the 3 phases of human sexual response. J Clin Psychiatry 2001;62(3):147–8.
15. Stahl SM. The psychopharmacology of sex, Part 1: Neurotransmitters and the 3 phases of the human sexual response. J Clin Psychiatry 2001;62(2):80–1.
16. Just MJ. The influence of atypical antipsychotic drugs on sexual function. Neuropsychiatr Dis Treat 2015;11:1655–61.

17. Atlantis E, Sullivan T. Bidirectional association between depression and sexual dysfunction: a systematic review and meta-analysis. J Sex Med 2012;9(6): 1497–507.

18. Kennedy SH, Dickens SE, Eisfeld BS, et al. Sexual dysfunction before antidepressant therapy in major depression. J Affect Disord 1999;56(2–3):201–8.

19. Yang JC, Park K, Eun SJ, et al. Assessment of cerebrocortical areas associated with sexual arousal in depressive women using functional MR imaging. J Sex Med 2008;5(3):602–9.

20. Perelman MA. The sexual tipping point: a mind/body model for sexual medicine. J Sex Med 2009;6(3):629–32.

21. Bloemers J, van Rooij K, Poels S, et al. Toward personalized sexual medicine (part 1): integrating the "dual control model" into differential drug treatments for hypoactive sexual desire disorder and female sexual arousal disorder. J Sex Med 2013;10(3):791–809.

22. Freeman ME, Kanyicska B, Lerant A, et al. Prolactin: structure, function, and regulation of secretion. Physiol Rev 2000;80(4):1523–631.

23. Hyyppa M, Rinne UK, Sonninen V. The activating effect of L-dopa treatment on sexual functions and its experimental background. Acta Neurol Scand 1970; 46(Suppl 43):223+.

24. Clayton AH, El Haddad S, Iluonakhamhe JP, et al. Sexual dysfunction associated with major depressive disorder and antidepressant treatment. Expert Opin Drug Saf 2014;13(10):1361–74.

25. Kleinberg DL, Davis JM, de Coster R, et al. Prolactin levels and adverse events in patients treated with risperidone. J Clin Psychopharmacol 1999;19(1):57–61.

26. Perez-Iglesias R, Mata I, Martínez-García O, et al. Long-term effect of haloperidol, olanzapine, and risperidone on plasma prolactin levels in patients with first-episode psychosis. J Clin Psychopharmacol 2012;32(6):804–8.

27. Berendsen HH, Jenck F, Broekkamp CL. Involvement of 5-HT1C-receptors in drug-induced penile erections in rats. Psychopharmacology (Berl) 1990; 101(1):57–61.

28. Ahlenius S, Larsson K, Svensson L, et al. Effects of a new type of 5-HT receptor agonist on male rat sexual behavior. Pharmacol Biochem Behav 1981;15(5): 785–92.

29. Ogawa S, Kudo S, Kitsunai Y, et al. Increase in oxytocin secretion at ejaculation in male. Clin Endocrinol (Oxf) 1980;13(1):95–7.

30. Murphy MR, Checkley SA, Seckl JR, et al. Naloxone inhibits oxytocin release at orgasm in man. J Clin Endocrinol Metab 1990;71(4):1056–8.

31. Rodriguez M, Castro R, Hernandez G, et al. Different roles of catecholaminergic and serotoninergic neurons of the medial forebrain bundle on male rat sexual behavior. Physiol Behav 1984;33(1):5–11.

32. Marson L, McKenna KE. The identification of a brainstem site controlling spinal sexual reflexes in male rats. Brain Res 1990;515(1–2):303–8.

33. Marberger H. The mechanisms of ejaculation. Basic Life Sci 1974;4(Pt. B): 99–110.

34. Truitt WA, Coolen LM. Identification of a potential ejaculation generator in the spinal cord. Science 2002;297(5586):1566–9.

35. Gitlin M. Sexual dysfunction with psychotropic drugs. Expert Opin Pharmacother 2003;4(12):2259–69.

36. Elnazer HY, Sampson A, Baldwin D. Lithium and sexual dysfunction: an under-researched area. Hum Psychopharmacol 2015;30(2):66–9.

37. Aizenberg D, Sigler M, Zemishlany Z, et al. Lithium and male sexual function in affective patients. Clin Neuropharmacol 1996;19(6):515–9.

38. Isojarvi JI, Löfgren E, Juntunen KS, et al. Effect of epilepsy and antiepileptic drugs on male reproductive health. Neurology 2004;62(2):247–53.

39. Isojarvi JI, Tauboll E, Herzog AG. Effect of antiepileptic drugs on reproductive endocrine function in individuals with epilepsy. CNS Drugs 2005;19(3):207–23.

40. Schneck CD, Thomas MR, Gundersen D. Sexual side effects associated with valproate. J Clin Psychopharmacol 2002;22(5):532–4.

41. Basson R, Rees P, Wang R, et al. Sexual function in chronic illness. J Sex Med 2010;7(1 Pt 2):374–88.

42. Penovich PE. The effects of epilepsy and its treatment on sexual and reproductive function. Epilepsia 2000;41(Suppl 2):S53–61.

43. Boora K, Chiappone K, Dubovsky SL. Oxcarbazepine-induced reversible anorgasmia and ejaculatory failure: a case report. Prim Care Companion J Clin Psychiatry 2009;11(4):173–4.

44. Calabro RS, Ferlazzo E, Italiano D, et al. Dose-dependent oxcarbazepine-related anorgasmia. Epilepsy Behav 2010;17(2):287–8.

45. Calabro RS, Italiano D, Pollicino P, et al. Oxcarbazepine-related retrograde ejaculation. Epilepsy Behav 2012;25(2):174–5.

46. Luef G, Kramer G, Stefan H. Oxcarbazepine treatment in male epilepsy patients improves pre-existing sexual dysfunction. Acta Neurol Scand 2009;119(2):94–9.

47. Brannon GE, Rolland PD. Anorgasmia in a patient with bipolar disorder type 1 treated with gabapentin. J Clin Psychopharmacol 2000;20(3):379–81.

48. Calabro RS, Bramanti P. Pregabalin-induced severe delayed ejaculation. Epilepsy Behav 2010;19(3):543.

49. Drabkin R, Calhoun L. Anorgasmia and withdrawal syndrome in a woman taking gabapentin. Can J Psychiatry 2003;48(2):125–6.

50. Grant AC, Oh H. Gabapentin-induced anorgasmia in women. Am J Psychiatry 2002;159(7):1247.

51. Hitiris N, Barrett JA, Brodie MJ. Erectile dysfunction associated with pregabalin add-on treatment in patients with partial seizures: five case reports. Epilepsy Behav 2006;8(2):418–21.

52. La Torre A, Giupponi G, Duffy D, et al. Sexual dysfunction related to psychotropic drugs: a critical review. Part III: mood stabilizers and anxiolytic drugs. Pharmacopsychiatry 2014;47(1):1–6.

53. Herzog AG, Drislane FW, Schomer DL, et al. Differential effects of antiepileptic drugs on sexual function and hormones in men with epilepsy. Neurology 2005;65(7):1016–20.

54. Herzog AG, Drislane FW, Schomer DL, et al. Differential effects of antiepileptic drugs on sexual function and reproductive hormones in men with epilepsy: interim analysis of a comparison between lamotrigine and enzyme-inducing antiepileptic drugs. Epilepsia 2004;45(7):764–8.

55. Stevenson JM, Bishop JR. Genetic determinants of selective serotonin reuptake inhibitor related sexual dysfunction. Pharmacogenomics 2014;15(14):1791–806.

56. Zourkova A, Hadasova E. Relationship between CYP 2D6 metabolic status and sexual dysfunction in paroxetine treatment. J Sex Marital Ther 2002;28(5):451–61.

57. Zourkova A, Ceskova E, Hadasová E, et al. Links among paroxetine-induced sexual dysfunctions, gender, and CYP2D6 activity. J Sex Marital Ther 2007;33(4):343–55.

58. Bly MJ, Bishop JR, Thomas KL, et al. P-glycoprotein (PGP) polymorphisms and sexual dysfunction in female patients with depression and SSRI-associated sexual side effects. J Sex Marital Ther 2013;39(3):280–8.

59. Zourkova A, Slanař O, Jarkovský J, et al. MDR1 in paroxetine-induced sexual dysfunction. J Sex Marital Ther 2013;39(1):71–8.

60. Bishop JR, Ellingrod VL, Akroush M, et al. The association of serotonin transporter genotypes and selective serotonin reuptake inhibitor (SSRI)-associated sexual side effects: possible relationship to oral contraceptives. Hum Psychopharmacol 2009;24(3):207–15.

61. Perlis RH, Mischoulon D, Smoller JW, et al. Serotonin transporter polymorphisms and adverse effects with fluoxetine treatment. Biol Psychiatry 2003;54(9): 879–83.

62. Strohmaier J, Wüst S, Uher R, et al. Sexual dysfunction during treatment with serotonergic and noradrenergic antidepressants: clinical description and the role of the 5-HTTLPR. World J Biol Psychiatry 2011;12(7):528–38.

63. Safarinejad MR. Analysis of association between the 5-HTTLPR and STin2 polymorphisms in the serotonin-transporter gene and clinical response to a selective serotonin reuptake inhibitor (sertraline) in patients with premature ejaculation. BJU Int 2010;105(1):73–8.

64. Janssen PK, Zwinderman AH, Olivier B, et al. Serotonin transporter promoter region (5-HTTLPR) polymorphism is not associated with paroxetine-induced ejaculation delay in Dutch men with lifelong premature ejaculation. Korean J Urol 2014;55(2):129–33.

65. Garfield LD, Dixon D, Nowotny P, et al. Common selective serotonin reuptake inhibitor side effects in older adults associated with genetic polymorphisms in the serotonin transporter and receptors: data from a randomized controlled trial. Am J Geriatr Psychiatry 2014;22(10):971–9.

66. Bishop JR, Moline J, Ellingrod VL, et al. Serotonin 2A -1438 G/A and G-protein Beta3 subunit C825T polymorphisms in patients with depression and SSRI-associated sexual side-effects. Neuropsychopharmacology 2006;31(10): 2281–8.

67. Liang CS, Ho PS, Chiang KT, et al. 5-HT2A receptor -1438 G/A polymorphism and serotonergic antidepressant-induced sexual dysfunction in male patients with major depressive disorder: a prospective exploratory study. J Sex Med 2012;9(8):2009–16.

68. Masiran R, Sidi H, Mohamed Z, et al. Association between 5HT2A polymorphism and selective serotonin re-uptake inhibitor (SSRI)-induced sexual desire disorder (SDD) among Malaysian women. Asia Pac Psychiatry 2013;5(Suppl 1):41–9.

69. Zou YF, Wang Y, Liu P, et al. Association of brain-derived neurotrophic factor genetic Val66Met polymorphism with severity of depression, efficacy of fluoxetine and its side effects in Chinese major depressive patients. Neuropsychobiology 2010;61(2):71–8.

70. Perlis RH, Laje G, Smoller JW, et al. Genetic and clinical predictors of sexual dysfunction in citalopram-treated depressed patients. Neuropsychopharmacology 2009;34(7):1819–28.

71. Bishop JR, Chae SS, Patel S, et al. Pharmacogenetics of glutamate system genes and SSRI-associated sexual dysfunction. Psychiatry Res 2012;199(1): 74–6.

72. Knegtering H, van der Moolen AE, Castelein S, et al. What are the effects of antipsychotics on sexual dysfunctions and endocrine functioning? Psychoneuroendocrinology 2003;28(Suppl 2):109–23.

73. Haberfellner EM. A review of the assessment of antidepressant-induced sexual dysfunction used in randomized, controlled clinical trials. Pharmacopsychiatry 2007;40(5):173–82.

74. La Torre A, Conca A, Duffy D, et al. Sexual dysfunction related to psychotropic drugs: a critical review part II: antipsychotics. Pharmacopsychiatry 2013;46(6): 201–8.

75. Monteiro WO, Noshirvani HF, Marks IM, et al. Anorgasmia from clomipramine in obsessive-compulsive disorder. A controlled trial. Br J Psychiatry 1987;151: 107–12.

76. Waldinger MD, Zwinderman AH, Olivier B. On-demand treatment of premature ejaculation with clomipramine and paroxetine: a randomized, double-blind fixed-dose study with stopwatch assessment. Eur Urol 2004;46(4):510–5 [discussion: 516].

77. Rosen RC, Lane RM, Menza M. Effects of SSRIs on sexual function: a critical review. J Clin Psychopharmacol 1999;19(1):67–85.

78. Gregorian RS, Golden KA, Bahce A, et al. Antidepressant-induced sexual dysfunction. Ann Pharmacother 2002;36(10):1577–89.

79. Clayton AH, Pradko JF, Croft HA, et al. Prevalence of sexual dysfunction among newer antidepressants. J Clin Psychiatry 2002;63(4):357–66.

80. Ashton AK, Mahmood A, Iqbal F. Improvements in SSRI/SNRI-induced sexual dysfunction by switching to escitalopram. J Sex Marital Ther 2005;31(3):257–62.

81. La Torre A, Giupponi G, Duffy D, et al. Sexual dysfunction related to psychotropic drugs: a critical review–part I: antidepressants. Pharmacopsychiatry 2013; 46(5):191–9.

82. Clayton A, Kornstein S, Prakash A, et al. Changes in sexual functioning associated with duloxetine, escitalopram, and placebo in the treatment of patients with major depressive disorder. J Sex Med 2007;4(4 Pt 1):917–29.

83. Gelenberg AJ, McGahuey C, Laukes C, et al. Mirtazapine substitution in SSRI-induced sexual dysfunction. J Clin Psychiatry 2000;61(5):356–60.

84. Wade A, Crawford GM, Angus M, et al. A randomized, double-blind, 24-week study comparing the efficacy and tolerability of mirtazapine and paroxetine in depressed patients in primary care. Int Clin Psychopharmacol 2003;18(3): 133–41.

85. Gardner EA, Johnston JA. Bupropion–an antidepressant without sexual pathophysiological action. J Clin Psychopharmacol 1985;5(1):24–9.

86. Dobkin RD, Menza M, Marin H, et al. Bupropion improves sexual functioning in depressed minority women: an open-label switch study. J Clin Psychopharmacol 2006;26(1):21–6.

87. Jacobsen PL, Clayton AH, Mahableshwarkar AR, et al. The effect of vortioxetine on sexual dysfunction in adults with major depressive disorder or generalized anxiety disorder. ASCP Meeting. Hollywood, FL, May 28, 2014.

88. Jacobsen PL, Mahableshwarkar AR, Chen Y, et al. Effect of vortioxetine vs. escitalopram on sexual functioning in adults with well-treated major depressive disorder experiencing SSRI-induced sexual dysfunction. J Sex Med 2015; 12(10):2036–48.

89. Yeragani VK, Gershon S. Priapism related to phenelzine therapy. N Engl J Med 1987;317(2):117–8.

90. Culpepper L, Kovalick LJ. A review of the literature on the selegiline transdermal system: an effective and well-tolerated monoamine oxidase inhibitor for the treatment of depression. Prim Care Companion J Clin Psychiatry 2008;10(1): 25–30.

91. Gartrell N. Increased libido in women receiving trazodone. Am J Psychiatry 1986;143(6):781–2.
92. Sullivan G. Increased libido in three men treated with trazodone. J Clin Psychiatry 1988;49(5):202–3.
93. Clayton AH, Kennedy SH, Edwards JB, et al. The effect of vilazodone on sexual function during the treatment of major depressive disorder. J Sex Med 2013; 10(10):2465–76.
94. Reis RM, de Angelo AG, Sakamoto AC, et al. Altered sexual and reproductive functions in epileptic men taking carbamazepine. J Sex Med 2013;10(2):493–9.
95. Elia J, Imbrogno N, Delfino M, et al. Retrograde ejaculation and abnormal hormonal profile in a subject under treatment with valproate and phenytoin. Arch Ital Urol Androl 2010;82(4):193–4.
96. Kristensen E, Jorgensen P. Sexual function in lithium-treated manic-depressive patients. Pharmacopsychiatry 1987;20(4):165–7.
97. Ghadirian AM, Annable L, Belanger MC. Lithium, benzodiazepines, and sexual function in bipolar patients. Am J Psychiatry 1992;149(6):801–5.
98. Marquez M, Arenoso H, Caruso N. Efficacy of alprazolam sublingual tablets in the treatment of the acute phase of panic disorders. Actas Esp Psiquiatr 2011;39(2):88–94.
99. Cutler AJ. Sexual dysfunction and antipsychotic treatment. Psychoneuroendocrinology 2003;28(Suppl 1):69–82.
100. Kotin J, Wilbert DE, Verburg D, et al. Thioridazine and sexual dysfunction. Am J Psychiatry 1976;133(1):82–5.
101. Compton MT, Miller AH. Priapism associated with conventional and atypical antipsychotic medications: a review. J Clin Psychiatry 2001;62(5):362–6.
102. Serretti A, Chiesa A. A meta-analysis of sexual dysfunction in psychiatric patients taking antipsychotics. Int Clin Psychopharmacol 2011;26(3):130–40.
103. Crawford AM, Beasley CM Jr, Tollefson GD. The acute and long-term effect of olanzapine compared with placebo and haloperidol on serum prolactin concentrations. Schizophr Res 1997;26(1):41–54.
104. Knegtering H, Boks M, Blijd C, et al. A randomized open-label comparison of the impact of olanzapine versus risperidone on sexual functioning. J Sex Marital Ther 2006;32(4):315–26.
105. Kelly DL, Conley RR. A randomized double-blind 12-week study of quetiapine, risperidone or fluphenazine on sexual functioning in people with schizophrenia. Psychoneuroendocrinology 2006;31(3):340–6.
106. Montejo AL, Majadas S, Rico-Villademoros F, et al. Frequency of sexual dysfunction in patients with a psychotic disorder receiving antipsychotics. J Sex Med 2010;7(10):3404–13.
107. Bobes J, Garc A-Portilla MP, Rejas J, et al. Frequency of sexual dysfunction and other reproductive side-effects in patients with schizophrenia treated with risperidone, olanzapine, quetiapine, or haloperidol: the results of the EIRE study. J Sex Marital Ther 2003;29(2):125–47.
108. Nakonezny PA, Byerly MJ, Rush AJ. The relationship between serum prolactin level and sexual functioning among male outpatients with schizophrenia or schizoaffective disorder: a randomized double-blind trial of risperidone vs. quetiapine. J Sex Marital Ther 2007;33(3):203–16.
109. Byerly MJ, Nakonezny PA, Rush AJ. Sexual functioning associated with quetiapine switch vs. risperidone continuation in outpatients with schizophrenia or schizoaffective disorder: a randomized double-blind pilot trial. Psychiatry Res 2008;159(1–2):115–20.

110. Dossenbach M, Dyachkova Y, Pirildar S, et al. Effects of atypical and typical antipsychotic treatments on sexual function in patients with schizophrenia: 12-month results from the Intercontinental Schizophrenia Outpatient Health Outcomes (IC-SOHO) study. Eur Psychiatry 2006;21(4):251–8.

111. Ucok A, Incesu C, Aker T, et al. Sexual dysfunction in patients with schizophrenia on antipsychotic medication. Eur Psychiatry 2007;22(5):328–33.

112. Kerwin R, Millet B, Herman E, et al. A multicentre, randomized, naturalistic, open-label study between aripiprazole and standard of care in the management of community-treated schizophrenic patients Schizophrenia Trial of Aripiprazole: (STAR) study. Eur Psychiatry 2007;22(7):433–43.

113. Montejo AL, Rico-Villademoros F, Spanish Working Group for the Study of Psychotropic-Related Sexual Dysfunction. Changes in sexual function for outpatients with schizophrenia or other psychotic disorders treated with ziprasidone in clinical practice settings: a 3-month prospective, observational study. J Clin Psychopharmacol 2008;28(5):568–70.

114. Clayton AH, Baker RA, Sheehan JJ, et al. Comparison of adjunctive use of aripiprazole with bupropion or selective serotonin reuptake inhibitors/serotonin-norepinephrine reuptake inhibitors: analysis of patients beginning adjunctive treatment in a 52-week, open-label study. BMC Res Notes 2014;7:459.

115. Berwaerts J, Cleton A, Rossenu S, et al. A comparison of serum prolactin concentrations after administration of paliperidone extended-release and risperidone tablets in patients with schizophrenia. J Psychopharmacol 2010;24(7):1011–8.

116. Montalvo I, Ortega L, López X, et al. Changes in prolactin levels and sexual function in young psychotic patients after switching from long-acting injectable risperidone to paliperidone palmitate. Int Clin Psychopharmacol 2013;28(1):46–9.

117. Shiloh R, Weizman A, Weizer N, et al. Risperidone-induced retrograde ejaculation. Am J Psychiatry 2001;158(4):650.

118. Serretti A, Chiesa A. Sexual side effects of pharmacological treatment of psychiatric diseases. Clin Pharmacol Ther 2011;89(1):142–7.

119. Hummer M, Kemmler G, Kurz M, et al. Sexual disturbances during clozapine and haloperidol treatment for schizophrenia. Am J Psychiatry 1999;156(4):631–3.

120. Deschenes S, Courtois F, Lafond J. Potential side effects of clozapine on the sexual function of schizophrenic men. J Sex Educ Ther 2001;26:332–9.

121. Freeman SA. Iloperidone-induced retrograde ejaculation. Int Clin Psychopharmacol 2013;28(3):156.

122. Cakin-Memik N, Yildiz O, Sişmanlar SG, et al. Priapism associated with methylphenidate: a case report. Turk J Pediatr 2010;52(4):430–4.

123. Oncu B, Colak B, Er O. Methylphenidate-induced spontaneous ejaculation. Ther Adv Psychopharmacol 2015;5(1):59–61.

124. Coskun M, Zoroglu S. A report of two cases of sexual side effects with OROS methylphenidate. J Child Adolesc Psychopharmacol 2009;19(4):477–9.

125. Taylor MJ, Rudkin L, Bullemor-Day P, et al. Strategies for managing sexual dysfunction induced by antidepressant medication. Cochrane Database Syst Rev 2013;(5):CD003382.

126. Nurnberg HG, Levine PE. Spontaneous remission of MAOI-induced anorgasmia. Am J Psychiatry 1987;144(6):805–7.

127. Reimherr FW, Chouinard G, Cohn CK, et al. Antidepressant efficacy of sertraline: a double-blind, placebo- and amitriptyline-controlled, multicenter comparison

study in outpatients with major depression. J Clin Psychiatry 1990;51(Suppl B): 18–27.

128. Segraves RT, Kavoussi R, Hughes AR, et al. Evaluation of sexual functioning in depressed outpatients: a double-blind comparison of sustained-release bupropion and sertraline treatment. J Clin Psychopharmacol 2000;20(2):122–8.

129. Ashton AK, Rosen RC. Bupropion as an antidote for serotonin reuptake inhibitor-induced sexual dysfunction. J Clin Psychiatry 1998;59(3):112–5.

130. Rothschild AJ. Selective serotonin reuptake inhibitor-induced sexual dysfunction: efficacy of a drug holiday. Am J Psychiatry 1995;152(10):1514–6.

131. Ferguson JM, Shrivastava RK, Stahl SM, et al. Reemergence of sexual dysfunction in patients with major depressive disorder: double-blind comparison of nefazodone and sertraline. J Clin Psychiatry 2001;62(1):24–9.

132. Lorenz TA, Meston CM. Acute exercise improves physical sexual arousal in women taking antidepressants. Ann Behav Med 2012;43(3):352–61.

133. Lorenz TA, Meston CM. Exercise improves sexual function in women taking antidepressants: results from a randomized crossover trial. Depress Anxiety 2014; 31(3):188–95.

134. Labbate LA, Croft HA, Oleshansky MA. Antidepressant-related erectile dysfunction: management via avoidance, switching antidepressants, antidotes, and adaptation. J Clin Psychiatry 2003;64(Suppl 10):11–9.

135. Montejo AL, Deakin JF, Gaillard R, et al. Better sexual acceptability of agomelatine (25 and 50 mg) compared to escitalopram (20 mg) in healthy volunteers. A 9-week, placebo-controlled study using the PRSexDQ scale. J Psychopharmacol 2015;29(10):1119–28.

136. Baldwin DS, Loft H, Dragheim M. A randomised, double-blind, placebo controlled, duloxetine-referenced, fixed-dose study of three dosages of Lu AA21004 in acute treatment of major depressive disorder (MDD). Eur Neuropsychopharmacol 2012;22(7):482–91.

137. Khan A, Cutler AJ, Kajdasz DK, et al. A randomized, double-blind, placebo-controlled, 8-week study of vilazodone, a serotonergic agent for the treatment of major depressive disorder. J Clin Psychiatry 2011;72(4):441–7.

138. Werneke U, Northey S, Bhugra D. Antidepressants and sexual dysfunction. Acta Psychiatr Scand 2006;114(6):384–97.

139. Montgomery SA, Baldwin DS, Riley A. Antidepressant medications: a review of the evidence for drug-induced sexual dysfunction. J Affect Disord 2002;69(1–3): 119–40.

140. Fava M, Rankin M. Sexual functioning and SSRIs. J Clin Psychiatry 2002; 63(Suppl 5):13–6 [discussion: 23–5].

141. Williams VS, Baldwin DS, Hogue SL, et al. Estimating the prevalence and impact of antidepressant-induced sexual dysfunction in 2 European countries: a cross-sectional patient survey. J Clin Psychiatry 2006;67(2):204–10.

142. Kennedy SH, Fulton KA, Bagby RM, et al. Sexual function during bupropion or paroxetine treatment of major depressive disorder. Can J Psychiatry 2006;51(4): 234–42.

143. Kennedy SH, Rizvi S, Fulton K, et al. A double-blind comparison of sexual functioning, antidepressant efficacy, and tolerability between agomelatine and venlafaxine XR. J Clin Psychopharmacol 2008;28(3):329–33.

144. Modell JG, Katholi CR, Modell JD, et al. Comparative sexual side effects of bupropion, fluoxetine, paroxetine, and sertraline. Clin Pharmacol Ther 1997;61(4): 476–87.

145. Dhillon S, Yang LP, Curran MP. Bupropion: a review of its use in the management of major depressive disorder. Drugs 2008;68(5):653–89.
146. Clayton AH, Croft HA, Horrigan JP, et al. Bupropion extended release compared with escitalopram: effects on sexual functioning and antidepressant efficacy in 2 randomized, double-blind, placebo-controlled studies. J Clin Psychiatry 2006; 67(5):736–46.
147. Coleman CC, King BR, Bolden-Watson C, et al. A placebo-controlled comparison of the effects on sexual functioning of bupropion sustained release and fluoxetine. Clin Ther 2001;23(7):1040–58.
148. Walker PW, Cole JO, Gardner EA, et al. Improvement in fluoxetine-associated sexual dysfunction in patients switched to bupropion. J Clin Psychiatry 1993; 54(12):459–65.
149. Croft H, Settle E Jr, Houser T, et al. A placebo-controlled comparison of the antidepressant efficacy and effects on sexual functioning of sustained-release bupropion and sertraline. Clin Ther 1999;21(4):643–58.
150. Coleman CC, Cunningham LA, Foster VJ, et al. Sexual dysfunction associated with the treatment of depression: a placebo-controlled comparison of bupropion sustained release and sertraline treatment. Ann Clin Psychiatry 1999;11(4): 205–15.
151. Thase ME, Clayton AH, Haight BR, et al. A double-blind comparison between bupropion XL and venlafaxine XR: sexual functioning, antidepressant efficacy, and tolerability. J Clin Psychopharmacol 2006;26(5):482–8.
152. Gartlehner G, Hansen RA, Morgan LC, et al. Comparative benefits and harms of second-generation antidepressants for treating major depressive disorder: an updated meta-analysis. Ann Intern Med 2011;155(11):772–85.
153. Clayton AH, Montejo AL. Major depressive disorder, antidepressants, and sexual dysfunction. J Clin Psychiatry 2006;67(Suppl 6):33–7.
154. Versiani M, Moreno R, Ramakers-van Moorsel CJ, et al. Comparison of the effects of mirtazapine and fluoxetine in severely depressed patients. CNS Drugs 2005;19(2):137–46.
155. Ozmenler NK, Karlidere T, Bozkurt A, et al. Mirtazapine augmentation in depressed patients with sexual dysfunction due to selective serotonin reuptake inhibitors. Hum Psychopharmacol 2008;23(4):321–6.
156. Ravindran LN, Eisfeld BS, Kennedy SH. Combining mirtazapine and duloxetine in treatment-resistant depression improves outcomes and sexual function. J Clin Psychopharmacol 2008;28(1):107–8.
157. Clayton AH, Gommoll C, Chen D, et al. Sexual dysfunction during treatment of major depressive disorder with vilazodone, citalopram, or placebo: results from a phase IV clinical trial. Int Clin Psychopharmacol 2015;30(4):216–23.
158. Citrome L. Vilazodone for major depressive disorder: a systematic review of the efficacy and safety profile for this newly approved antidepressant - what is the number needed to treat, number needed to harm and likelihood to be helped or harmed? Int J Clin Pract 2012;66(4):356–68.
159. Robinson DS, Kajdasz DK, Gallipoli S, et al. A 1-year, open-label study assessing the safety and tolerability of vilazodone in patients with major depressive disorder. J Clin Psychopharmacol 2011;31(5):643–6.
160. Rickels K, Athanasiou M, Robinson DS, et al. Evidence for efficacy and tolerability of vilazodone in the treatment of major depressive disorder: a randomized, double-blind, placebo-controlled trial. J Clin Psychiatry 2009;70(3):326–33.

161. Sanchez C, Asin KE, Artigas F. Vortioxetine, a novel antidepressant with multimodal activity: review of preclinical and clinical data. Pharmacol Ther 2015; 145:43–57.

162. Clayton AH, Reddy S, Focht K, et al. An evaluation of sexual functioning in employed outpatients with major depressive disorder treated with desvenlafaxine 50 mg or placebo. J Sex Med 2013;10(3):768–76.

163. Clayton AH, Hwang E, Kornstein SG, et al. Effects of 50 and 100 mg desvenlafaxine versus placebo on sexual function in patients with major depressive disorder: a meta-analysis. Int Clin Psychopharmacol 2015;30(6):307–15.

164. Ferguson JM. The effects of antidepressants on sexual functioning in depressed patients: a review. J Clin Psychiatry 2001;62(Suppl 3):22–34.

165. Feiger A, Kiev A, Shrivastava RK, et al. Nefazodone versus sertraline in outpatients with major depression: focus on efficacy, tolerability, and effects on sexual function and satisfaction. J Clin Psychiatry 1996;57(Suppl 2):53–62.

166. Waldinger MD, Zwinderman AH, Olivier B. Antidepressants and ejaculation: a double-blind, randomized, placebo-controlled, fixed-dose study with paroxetine, sertraline, and nefazodone. J Clin Psychopharmacol 2001;21(3):293–7.

167. Kennedy SH, Eisfeld BS, Dickens SE, et al. Antidepressant-induced sexual dysfunction during treatment with moclobemide, paroxetine, sertraline, and venlafaxine. J Clin Psychiatry 2000;61(4):276–81.

168. Baldwin DS. Sexual dysfunction associated with antidepressant drugs. Expert Opin Drug Saf 2004;3(5):457–70.

169. Vanderkooy JD, Kennedy SH, Bagby RM. Antidepressant side effects in depression patients treated in a naturalistic setting: a study of bupropion, moclobemide, paroxetine, sertraline, and venlafaxine. Can J Psychiatry 2002;47(2): 174–80.

170. Ramasubbu R. Switching to moclobemide to reverse fluoxetine-induced sexual dysfunction in patients with depression. J Psychiatry Neurosci 1999;24(1): 45–50.

171. Philipp M, Kohnen R, Benkert O. A comparison study of moclobemide and doxepin in major depression with special reference to effects on sexual dysfunction. Int Clin Psychopharmacol 1993;7(3–4):149–53.

172. Clayton AH, Zajecka J, Ferguson JM, et al. Lack of sexual dysfunction with the selective noradrenaline reuptake inhibitor reboxetine during treatment for major depressive disorder. Int Clin Psychopharmacol 2003;18(3):151–6.

173. Langworth S, Bodlund O, Agren H. Efficacy and tolerability of reboxetine compared with citalopram: a double-blind study in patients with major depressive disorder. J Clin Psychopharmacol 2006;26(2):121–7.

174. Baldwin D, Bridgman K, Buis C. Resolution of sexual dysfunction during double-blind treatment of major depression with reboxetine or paroxetine. J Psychopharmacol 2006;20(1):91–6.

175. Mucci M. Reboxetine: a review of antidepressant tolerability. J Psychopharmacol 1997;11(4 Suppl):S33–7.

176. Khazaie H, Rezaie L, Rezaei Payam N, et al. Antidepressant-induced sexual dysfunction during treatment with fluoxetine, sertraline and trazodone; a randomized controlled trial. Gen Hosp Psychiatry 2015;37(1):40–5.

177. Atmaca M, Kuloglu M, Tezcan E, et al. Switching to tianeptine in patients with antidepressant-induced sexual dysfunction. Hum Psychopharmacol 2003; 18(4):277–80.

178. Michelson D, Bancroft J, Targum S, et al. Female sexual dysfunction associated with antidepressant administration: a randomized, placebo-controlled study of pharmacologic intervention. Am J Psychiatry 2000;157(2):239–43.

179. Baldwin DS, Palazzo MC, Masdrakis VG. Reduced treatment-emergent sexual dysfunction as a potential target in the development of new antidepressants. Depress Res Treat 2013;2013:256841.

180. Zajecka J. Strategies for the treatment of antidepressant-related sexual dysfunction. J Clin Psychiatry 2001;62(Suppl 3):35–43.

181. Safarinejad MR, Hosseini SY, Asgari MA, et al. A randomized, double-blind, placebo-controlled study of the efficacy and safety of bupropion for treating hypoactive sexual desire disorder in ovulating women. BJU Int 2010;106(6):832–9.

182. Segraves RT, Croft H, Kavoussi R, et al. Bupropion sustained release (SR) for the treatment of hypoactive sexual desire disorder (HSDD) in nondepressed women. J Sex Marital Ther 2001;27(3):303–16.

183. Safarinejad MR. The effects of the adjunctive bupropion on male sexual dysfunction induced by a selective serotonin reuptake inhibitor: a double-blind placebo-controlled and randomized study. BJU Int 2010;106(6):840–7.

184. Thase ME, Haight BR, Richard N, et al. Remission rates following antidepressant therapy with bupropion or selective serotonin reuptake inhibitors: a meta-analysis of original data from 7 randomized controlled trials. J Clin Psychiatry 2005;66(8):974–81.

185. Clayton AH, Warnock JK, Kornstein SG, et al. A placebo-controlled trial of bupropion SR as an antidote for selective serotonin reuptake inhibitor-induced sexual dysfunction. J Clin Psychiatry 2004;65(1):62–7.

186. DeBattista C, Solvason B, Poirier J, et al. A placebo-controlled, randomized, double-blind study of adjunctive bupropion sustained release in the treatment of SSRI-induced sexual dysfunction. J Clin Psychiatry 2005;66(7):844–8.

187. Masand PS, Ashton AK, Gupta S, et al. Sustained-release bupropion for selective serotonin reuptake inhibitor-induced sexual dysfunction: a randomized, double-blind, placebo-controlled, parallel-group study. Am J Psychiatry 2001; 158(5):805–7.

188. Safarinejad MR. Reversal of SSRI-induced female sexual dysfunction by adjunctive bupropion in menstruating women: a double-blind, placebo-controlled and randomized study. J Psychopharmacol 2011;25(3):370–8.

189. Nurnberg HG, Hensley PL, Gelenberg AJ, et al. Treatment of antidepressant-associated sexual dysfunction with sildenafil: a randomized controlled trial. JAMA 2003;289(1):56–64.

190. Fava M, Nurnberg HG, Seidman SN, et al. Efficacy and safety of sildenafil in men with serotonergic antidepressant-associated erectile dysfunction: results from a randomized, double-blind, placebo-controlled trial. J Clin Psychiatry 2006;67(2):240–6.

191. Nurnberg HG, Hensley PL, Heiman JR, et al. Sildenafil treatment of women with antidepressant-associated sexual dysfunction: a randomized controlled trial. JAMA 2008;300(4):395–404.

192. Evliyaoglu Y, Yelsel K, Kobaner M, et al. Efficacy and tolerability of tadalafil for treatment of erectile dysfunction in men taking serotonin reuptake inhibitors. Urology 2011;77(5):1137–41.

193. Michelson D, Kociban K, Tamura R, et al. Mirtazapine, yohimbine or olanzapine augmentation therapy for serotonin reuptake-associated female sexual dysfunction: a randomized, placebo controlled trial. J Psychiatr Res 2002;36(3):147–52.

194. Farah A. Relief of SSRI-induced sexual dysfunction with mirtazapine treatment. J Clin Psychiatry 1999;60(4):260–1.

195. Landen M, Eriksson E, Agren H, et al. Effect of buspirone on sexual dysfunction in depressed patients treated with selective serotonin reuptake inhibitors. J Clin Psychopharmacol 1999;19(3):268–71.

196. Norden M. Buspirone treatment of sexual dysfunction associated with selective serotonin reuptake inhibitors. Depression 1994;2:109–12.

197. Gaynes BN, Warden D, Trivedi MH, et al. What did STAR*D teach us? Results from a large-scale, practical, clinical trial for patients with depression. Psychiatr Serv 2009;60(11):1439–45.

198. Javanbakht A. As-needed use of cyproheptadine for treatment of selective serotonin reuptake inhibitor-related female anorgasmia. J Clin Psychopharmacol 2015;35(1):91–3.

199. McCormick S, Olin J, Brotman AW. Reversal of fluoxetine-induced anorgasmia by cyproheptadine in two patients. J Clin Psychiatry 1990;51(9):383–4.

200. Cohen AJ. Fluoxetine-induced yawning and anorgasmia reversed by cyproheptadine treatment. J Clin Psychiatry 1992;53(5):174.

201. Arnott S, Nutt D. Successful treatment of fluvoxamine-induced anorgasmia by cyproheptadine. Br J Psychiatry 1994;164(6):838–9.

202. Feder R. Reversal of antidepressant activity of fluoxetine by cyproheptadine in three patients. J Clin Psychiatry 1991;52(4):163–4.

203. Aukst-Margetic B, Margetic B. An open-label series using loratadine for the treatment of sexual dysfunction associated with selective serotonin reuptake inhibitors. Prog Neuropsychopharmacol Biol Psychiatry 2005;29(5):754–6.

204. Balogh S, Hendricks SE, Kang J. Treatment of fluoxetine-induced anorgasmia with amantadine. J Clin Psychiatry 1992;53(6):212–3.

205. Shrivastava RK, Shrivastava S, Overweg N, et al. Amantadine in the treatment of sexual dysfunction associated with selective serotonin reuptake inhibitors. J Clin Psychopharmacol 1995;15(1):83–4.

206. Balon R. Intermittent amantadine for fluoxetine-induced anorgasmia. J Sex Marital Ther 1996;22(4):290–2.

207. Clayton AH, McGarvey EL, Warnock J, et al. Bupropion SR as an antidote to SSRI-induced sexual dysfunction. 40th Annual NCDEU Meeting. National Institute of Mental Health. New Orleans, LA, 2001. Poster 169.

208. Bernik M, Vieira AH, Nunes PV. Bethanecol chloride for treatment of clomipramine-induced orgasmic dysfunction in males. Rev Hosp Clin Fac Med Sao Paulo 2004;59(6):357–60.

209. Gross MD. Reversal by bethanechol of sexual dysfunction caused by anticholinergic antidepressants. Am J Psychiatry 1982;139(9):1193–4.

210. Segraves RT. Reversal by bethanechol of imipramine-induced ejaculatory dysfunction. Am J Psychiatry 1987;144(9):1243–4.

211. Jespersen S, Berk M, Van Wyk C, et al. A pilot randomized, double-blind, placebo-controlled study of granisetron in the treatment of sexual dysfunction in women associated with antidepressant use. Int Clin Psychopharmacol 2004; 19(3):161–4.

212. Nelson EB, Shah VN, Welge JA, et al. A placebo-controlled, crossover trial of granisetron in SRI-induced sexual dysfunction. J Clin Psychiatry 2001;62(6): 469–73.

213. Dording CM, Mischoulon D, Shyu I, et al. SAMe and sexual functioning. Eur Psychiatry 2012;27(6):451–4.

214. Kang BJ, Lee SJ, Kim MD, et al. A placebo-controlled, double-blind trial of Ginkgo biloba for antidepressant-induced sexual dysfunction. Hum Psychopharmacol 2002;17(6):279–84.
215. Wheatley D. Triple-blind, placebo-controlled trial of Ginkgo biloba in sexual dysfunction due to antidepressant drugs. Hum Psychopharmacol 2004;19(8):545–8.
216. Farnia V, Hojatitabar S, Shakeri J, et al. Adjuvant Rosa Damascena has a Small Effect on SSRI-induced Sexual Dysfunction in Female Patients Suffering from MDD. Pharmacopsychiatry 2015;48(4–5):156–63.
217. Farnia V, Shirzadifar M, Shakeri J, et al. Rosa damascena oil improves SSRI-induced sexual dysfunction in male patients suffering from major depressive disorders: results from a double-blind, randomized, and placebo-controlled clinical trial. Neuropsychiatr Dis Treat 2015;11:625–35.
218. Dording CM, Fisher L, Papakostas G, et al. A double-blind, randomized, pilot dose-finding study of maca root (*L. meyenii*) for the management of SSRI-induced sexual dysfunction. CNS Neurosci Ther 2008;14(3):182–91.
219. Dording CM, Schettler PJ, Dalton ED, et al. A double-blind placebo-controlled trial of maca root as treatment for antidepressant-induced sexual dysfunction in women. Evid Based Complement Alternat Med 2015;2015:949036.
220. Byerly MJ, Nakonezny PA, Bettcher BM, et al. Sexual dysfunction associated with second-generation antipsychotics in outpatients with schizophrenia or schizoaffective disorder: an empirical evaluation of olanzapine, risperidone, and quetiapine. Schizophr Res 2006;86(1–3):244–50.
221. Nagaraj AK, Pai NB, Rao S. A comparative study of sexual dysfunction involving risperidone, quetiapine, and olanzapine. Indian J Psychiatry 2009;51(4):265–71.
222. Bitter I, Basson BR, Dossenbach MR. Antipsychotic treatment and sexual functioning in first-time neuroleptic-treated schizophrenic patients. Int Clin Psychopharmacol 2005;20(1):19–21.
223. Kinon BJ, Ahl J, Liu-Seifert H, et al. Improvement in hyperprolactinemia and reproductive comorbidities in patients with schizophrenia switched from conventional antipsychotics or risperidone to olanzapine. Psychoneuroendocrinology 2006;31(5):577–88.
224. Schmidt HM, Hagen M, Kriston L, et al. Management of sexual dysfunction due to antipsychotic drug therapy. Cochrane Database Syst Rev 2012;(11):CD003546.
225. Mir A, Shivakumar K, Williamson RJ, et al. Change in sexual dysfunction with aripiprazole: a switching or add-on study. J Psychopharmacol 2008;22(3):244–53.
226. Gopalakrishnan R, Jacob KS, Kuruvilla A, et al. Sildenafil in the treatment of antipsychotic-induced erectile dysfunction: a randomized, double-blind, placebo-controlled, flexible-dose, two-way crossover trial. Am J Psychiatry 2006;163(3):494–9.

Adverse Effects in the Pharmacologic Management of Bipolar Disorder During Pregnancy

CrossMark

Charlotte S. Hogan, MD[a], Marlene P. Freeman, MD[b],*

KEYWORDS

- Pregnancy • Bipolar disorder • Adverse effects • Lithium • Anticonvulsant
- Antipsychotic

KEY POINTS

- Bipolar disorder is associated with maternal and fetal risks independent of medication exposure.
- Management of bipolar disorder during pregnancy often requires medication with potential teratogenic risks or inadequately characterized reproductive safety profiles.
- Reproductive safety data should be considered when prescribing medication for all women of childbearing potential.
- Lithium is associated with risks during pregnancy and requires careful monitoring, yet may be a first-line treatment for some women.
- Valproate is contraindicated during pregnancy because of high risk for numerous adverse effects.
- Atypical antipsychotics are the subject of a growing body of literature that appears largely reassuring.

INTRODUCTION

Bipolar disorder is common (worldwide lifetime prevalence is 2.4%)[1] and associated with significant disability, morbidity, and mortality.[2–4] The age of onset is usually between the teenage years and early 40s,[5] thereby frequently affecting women of childbearing age. Pregnancy and the postpartum period are times of particular

Dr C.S. Hogan has nothing to disclose.
Advisory Boards: Sunovion, Takeda, JDS Therapeutics, JayMac Pharmaceuticals, Research Support (investigator, initiated study): Takeda (IISR VOR-IIT-0006), Janssen/Johnson & Johnson: Independent Data Safety and Monitoring Committee, GOED medical editing (Dr M.P. Freeman).

[a] Department of Psychiatry, Massachusetts General Hospital, Warren 605, 55 Fruit Street, Boston, MA 02114, USA; [b] Department of Psychiatry, Massachusetts General Hospital, Simches 2, 185 Cambridge Street, Boston, MA 02114, USA
* Corresponding author.
E-mail address: mfreeman@mgh.harvard.edu

Psychiatr Clin N Am 39 (2016) 465–475
http://dx.doi.org/10.1016/j.psc.2016.04.007
0193-953X/16/$ – see front matter © 2016 Elsevier Inc. All rights reserved.

vulnerability for women with bipolar disorder.[6,7] Pregnancy does not appear to have a protective effect against new or worsening bipolar illness, and it may increase the risk of depressive symptoms.[8] It has been suggested that when mood-stabilizing medications are discontinued during pregnancy, especially if this is done abruptly, there is a greater risk of recurrence (85.5%) than when treatment is continued (37%).[8] The postpartum period has been clearly associated with a further significant elevation in the risk of mood episodes in women with bipolar disorder.[9,10]

Importantly, bipolar disorder is associated with maternal and fetal risks independent of medication exposure and should be thought of as a separate fetal "exposure" during pregnancy. Fetal risks related to symptomatic maternal bipolar disorder include microcephaly, small gestational age, prematurity, low Apgar scores, and increased admissions to the neonatal intensive care unit.[11–13] In addition to the morbidity of the disorder itself, maternal bipolar disorder has been associated with obstetric complications, lack of engagement with prenatal care, and increased substance abuse during pregnancy.[13,14] The postpartum period is also associated with significant risk in the setting of untreated bipolar illness. Postpartum psychosis, for example, is a psychiatric emergency that occurs in 1 to 2/1000 childbearing women and is associated with bipolar disorder in 72% to 88% of cases.[15] Risk is also inherent in pregnancy itself. The risk of major congenital malformations (MCM) in the general US population is about 3%.[16]

Therefore, it is important to prioritize mood stability when managing bipolar disorder during pregnancy. Maintenance of euthymia often involves medications that have potential teratogenic risks or may involve inadequately characterized reproductive safety profiles. Women with bipolar disorder who are planning pregnancy, therefore, face challenging decisions about their treatment; careful risk-benefit discussions are necessary. With the goal of further informing these discussions, this article reviews the data currently available regarding medication safety in the management of bipolar disorder during pregnancy. This review focuses specifically on the medications with the strongest evidence base for use as mood stabilizers in bipolar disorder, specifically lithium, valproic acid, lamotrigine, carbamazepine, and antipsychotic medications.[17]

LITHIUM

Although lithium has been characterized as a teratogen, it is an important mood stabilizer to consider during pregnancy for women who are known to be lithium responders. Teratogenic risks associated with lithium have been well studied and well quantified. Specifically, lithium exposure during the first trimester has been linked to Ebstein anomaly, a displacement and malformation of the tricuspid valve that results in atrialization of the right ventricle, resulting in tricuspid regurgitation and usually requiring surgical repair.[18] In initial studies, the risk of this cardiovascular defect with lithium exposure was thought to be quite high; however, more recent cohort and case control studies demonstrated that the absolute risk is actually lower.[19] In the general population, Ebstein anomaly occurs in 1/20,000 live births; with first-trimester lithium exposure, the risk is estimated to be 1/1000 or lower.[20] Several other case control studies have not demonstrated a clear association between lithium exposure and Ebstein anomaly.[21] For some women treated with lithium, it may be reasonable to discontinue its use during the first trimester. For women with severe illness, it may be reasonable to continue lithium throughout pregnancy, despite the known but low absolute risk of malformations. Given remaining uncertainty about this risk, it is prudent to recommend that women taking lithium during their first trimester undergo a level II ultrasound and fetal echocardiography at 16 to 20 weeks' gestation to assess for cardiac malformation, in order to facilitate informed decision making about continuing the pregnancy as well as potential planning for neonatal surgical intervention.[22]

Adverse effects in the neonate that have been reported with late antenatal lithium use include cases of neonatal hypotonia, lethargy, and respiratory distress.[23] Other rare neonatal complications include diabetes insipidus, nephrotoxicity, hypothyroidism, arrhythmias, and hepatic dysfunction.[20,23,24] It may be possible to decrease the risk of these neonatal outcomes by discontinuing lithium 24 to 48 hours before planned deliveries, or at the onset of labor in spontaneous deliveries.[20] However, this strategy must be carefully considered, because the risk of postpartum relapse is high in women with bipolar disorder,[25] and it is not known whether briefly stopping lithium around delivery impacts risk of relapse.

Data on long-term neurodevelopmental outcomes in children exposed to lithium prenatally are sparse, although 2 small studies have not shown any motor or cognitive developmental anomalies in childhood.[26,27]

Notable potential maternal adverse effects of lithium during pregnancy include exacerbation of polyuria and polydipsia as well as increased nausea, weight gain, hypertension, and gestational diabetes.[22]

Because of pregnancy-related changes in vascular volumes and the glomerular filtration rate, lithium levels and mood need to be closely monitored throughout pregnancy, with many pregnant women experiencing clinically significant declines in lithium levels. Standard guidelines recommend that serum lithium levels and routine thyroid/renal function laboratory tests be drawn monthly from the 20th week of gestation and then weekly beginning 4 weeks before expected delivery.[28] Some women require an increased lithium dose during pregnancy[29]; however this should be based on clinical symptoms rather than specific serum levels. It is important to monitor for common conditions (eg, preeclampsia, hyperemesis gravidarum, diuretic use) that would predispose the patient to lithium toxicity.[20,30] After delivery, rapid postpartum diuresis and return of the pregravid glomerular filtration rate necessitate attention to hydration and reinstitution of the patient's prepregnancy lithium dose to avoid toxicity.[29]

Lithium is perhaps the psychotropic of greatest risk in breast-feeding, with its use during breast-feeding considered reasonable only in certain circumstances.[31] Lithium is excreted in breast milk, with the concentration of lithium in infant serum approximating one-quarter the concentration of lithium in maternal serum.[31] Infants breastfed by mothers taking lithium should be closely monitored, behaviorally and with periodic measurement of lithium level, thyroid stimulating hormone, and blood urea nitrogen/creatinine.[32] Given the risks of infant lithium exposure and the demands of frequent infant monitoring, as well as the potential threat to maternal mood stability posed by nighttime feedings, breast-feeding while on lithium therapy should only be recommended in cases of mothers with stable mood and demonstrated treatment adherence, healthy infants, and a collaborative pediatrician.[31]

ANTIEPILEPTIC DRUGS
Valproic Acid

Valproic acid administration during pregnancy carries a definite increase in risk of serious teratogenic as well as neurodevelopmental anomalies, and it is generally contraindicated both in pregnancy and in women of reproductive potential.[33] Prenatal valproate exposure results in greater than 9% risk of MCM.[34,35] Because of valproate's interference with folate metabolism, neural tube defects are common, occurring in 2% to 5% of valproate-exposed fetuses (20-fold greater than in the general population).[36]

The neural tube forms during the early weeks of pregnancy, and, therefore, valproate used before conception and before a woman is aware she is pregnant is of grave concern. Valproate use during pregnancy also increases the risks of craniofacial defects, oral clefts, cardiac defects, hypospadias, and polydactyly.[37,38] Infants exposed to valproate prenatally additionally have increased rates of hypoglycemia[39] and may experience a neonatal toxicity syndrome characterized by irritability, hypertonia, feeding problems, and low Apgar scores.[40]

Numerous recent studies also show a clear relationship between prenatal valproate exposure and neurocognitive developmental anomalies. These anomalies include significantly lower IQ, impaired cognition over several domains (memory/language/executive function), and poor adaptive functioning.[41,42] In addition, valproate exposure appears to increase risks of autism and attention deficit hyperactivity disorder.[42,43] Because the brain continues to develop throughout pregnancy, valproate should be avoided for the duration of pregnancy. Because of its associated risks in pregnancy and the high frequency of unplanned pregnancies, caution must also be used in prescribing valproate to women of childbearing age. Standard of care, in the authors' opinion, should dictate that young women have long-acting contraception before prescription of valproate.

Although valproate should generally be avoided in women of reproductive potential, there have not been specific data to raise concern about its use in breast-feeding. Because it is plasma protein–bound, it is excreted in low quantities in breast milk; concentrations in breast milk are 1% to 10% of the maternal serum valproate levels.[44] Although studies are few, major adverse events have not been reported.[45] Notably, immature hepatic metabolism results in a longer valproate half-life in newborns (47 hours) than adults (7–12 hours).[44] This raises concern for the theoretic risk of thrombocytopenia and hepatotoxicity in the infant, and monitoring is warranted.[45]

Lamotrigine

Lamotrigine, which has been well studied by several pregnancy registries, appears to be relatively safe during pregnancy. These registries have demonstrated that lamotrigine use during pregnancy is associated with a 2% to 5% risk of MCM, which is comparable to the general population.[34,35,46] In addition, despite earlier suspicions that lamotrigine increased risk for oral clefts, this association has not been observed in larger registries.[34,46] Risks of MCM may be dose-dependent,[35,47] and so, as with other medications during pregnancy, lamotrigine should be administered at the lowest therapeutic dose. Studies following children who were exposed prenatally to lamotrigine up to 6 years old have not demonstrated neurodevelopmental abnormalities.[41,48,49]

Lamotrigine metabolism is significantly affected by changes in estrogen levels because estrogen upregulates hepatic glucuronidation.[50] Lamotrigine adverse effects can, therefore, present when a woman discontinues oral contraception to prepare for pregnancy.[51] During pregnancy, lamotrigine levels decrease significantly, and the dose generally has to be increased throughout pregnancy in order to maintain therapeutic levels and avoid symptom relapse.[52]

Breast-feeding while on lamotrigine is considered reasonable with careful clinical monitoring. Although lamotrigine levels are measurable in infant serum with breast-feeding,[50] only one case of an adverse event related to this exposure has been reported: apnea in an infant breast-fed by a lamotrigine-toxic mother.[53] Immature hepatic metabolism in infants means that levels may be higher than in adults.[50]

Carbamazepine

Despite lower risks of MCM than valproic acid,[54] fetal exposure to carbamazepine is also of concern. Although low doses during pregnancy have not been demonstrated to clearly increase the risk of MCM above the general population, at higher doses (>1000 mg daily), carbamazepine is associated with elevated risk of MCM ranging from 5.3% to 7.7%.[35,47] There is an association between first-trimester carbamazepine exposure and spina bifida with an odds ratio of 2.6; data are less consistent for associations with oral clefts, hypospadias, and cardiovascular defects.[54] Exposure to carbamazepine also results in a small but statistically significant increase in risk of fetal growth restriction and decreased head circumference.[38,55]

In a dose-dependent manner, carbamazepine exposure may affect development of verbal skills, motor skills, and adaptive functioning in early childhood.[56]

Notably, carbamazepine increases the metabolism of oral contraceptives, which may lead to an unplanned pregnancy.[57] Like other psychotropics, carbamazepine is transmitted in breast milk. However, infant drug levels are generally low enough to be of minimal clinical concern.[58]

ANTIPSYCHOTICS
First-Generation Antipsychotics

As a class, first-generation antipsychotics (FGAs) have been used during pregnancy for decades, and there has been no definitive association identified between FGA administration and any increased rate or specific pattern of malformations.[59,60] However, large prospective studies assessing FGAs in pregnancy are limited. It has been suggested that the risk of MCM may be slightly increased with first-trimester exposure to low potency agents, whereas high-potency antipsychotics, such as haloperidol, perphenazine, trifluoperazine, and thiothixene, may be safer.[61] Although data are limited, FGA exposure has been associated with increased risks of low birth weight[62] and preterm delivery[63]; it is not clear, however, if these risks are due to the medication itself or to other risk factors in the population of women with disorders warranting antipsychotic use.

FGA exposure in utero has been associated with a syndrome in newborns characterized by restlessness, tremor, feeding difficulties, increased tone, dystonias, and parkinsonism, thought to represent neonatal extrapyramidal symptoms.[59,64] The US Food and Drug Administration issued a drug safety announcement in 2011 regarding this syndrome when 69 cases were identified after FGA or atypical antipsychotic use. Many of these cases involved polypharmacy, and the clinical significance is undetermined.[65] These symptoms are typically of short duration (2–6 days) and without long-term consequences.[66]

Long-term neurobehavioral outcomes have not been thoroughly or systematically studied. One large prospective cohort study did not demonstrate any difference in IQ at age 4 in children exposed to FGA compared with those who were not exposed.[67]

Safety data regarding breast-feeding while on FGA are limited, but generally reassuring. Drug levels in the breast milk are low at less than 3% of the maternal dose.[68]

Second-Generation Antipsychotics (Atypical Antipsychotics)

Second-generation antipsychotics (SGAs) are prescribed increasingly frequently, with a greater than 200% increase in the prescription of these medications between 2000 and 2011.[59] Despite this increasing use, until recently there have been relatively little data regarding their reproductive safety.

The first prospective study on the reproductive safety of SGAs did not show any differences in the rates of malformations between the group with first-trimester exposure to SGA (0.9%) and the control group (1.5%).[69] Another larger prospective study suggested the possibility of an increase in risk of septal heart defects in infants exposed to SGA during pregnancy compared with those not exposed (odds ratio 2.17).[70] The Australian National Register of Antipsychotic Medication in Pregnancy published early results of its ongoing prospective observational study, which were notable for somewhat high rates of MCM (5.6%), although this study lacked a control group.[71] An additional study did not find an increased risk of MCM with exposure to SGA, but did suggest that exposed infants were more likely to receive specialized neonatal care, particularly in the setting of maternal polypharmacy.[72] Finally, the National Pregnancy Registry for Atypical Antipsychotics also recently reported initial results from its prospective study, finding no significant difference between rates of major malformations in infants exposed to an SGA (1.4%) and a comparison group (1.1%).[73]

Overall, these studies are reassuring regarding the reproductive safety of SGAs; however, more data are required to definitively understand risks. In addition, the newest SGAs are underrepresented in these studies, and there are not sufficient data to comment on the reproductive safety of these newer agents.

SGA exposure during pregnancy appears to affect risk for abnormal birth weight in infants, with several studies demonstrating an increased risk of infants being large for gestational age[63,74] and others demonstrating potential risk for abnormally low birth weight.[75] Long-term neurobehavioral outcomes of SGA exposure during pregnancy have not been systematically studied.

Regarding maternal health, SGAs are well known to increase risk of weight gain and adverse metabolic conditions, such as insulin resistance and hyperlipidemia.[76] During pregnancy, these adverse effects of SGA administration translate into increased risk of excessive weight gain[77] and gestational diabetes, which is twice as common in women taking antipsychotic medication.[78,79] The degree to which these risks may be explained by mental illness as a confounding factor, however, is unknown.

Data regarding safety of breast-feeding while taking SGAs are lacking. Olanzapine, risperidone, and quetiapine have received some study, although very few cases are represented in the literature, and it appears that plasma drug levels in breast-fed infants are low.[80–82] If women breast-feed while using an SGA, infants should be monitored closely for sedation and other potential adverse effects.[83]

DISCUSSION

This growing body of reproductive safety data for the pharmacologic management of bipolar disorder during pregnancy has several implications. Women with bipolar disorder planning pregnancy require careful counseling and education about these medications, in addition to being informed about the limitations of current available data and the known risks of nontreatment. This clinical scenario is not uncommon, with an estimated 60% of women around the world with severe mental illness having children.[84] Qualitative data exploring the experiences of women with severe mental illness, including bipolar disorder, also identify a common theme of motherhood being both rewarding and central to the individual's life, in addition to being a protective factor that promotes recovery.[84] Supporting healthy pregnancy and successful transition to motherhood, where possible, is an important role of the psychiatrist.

In addition, prescribers must take this data into account in the management of any woman with bipolar disorder of childbearing age given high rates of unplanned pregnancies. In 2011, for example, 45% of pregnancies in the United States were unintended.[85] This rate may be even higher among women with major mental illness. In women with bipolar disorder specifically, one study found that only 33% of pregnancies were planned, and there was a trend toward younger age at first pregnancy compared with a control group of women without bipolar disorder.[86] Consideration of pregnancy safety data, and attention to contraceptive care if appropriate, must be a part of the management of bipolar disorder in all women with bipolar disorder until they are beyond the reproductive years.

This review specifically covered potential adverse effects of medications used in the management of bipolar disorder during pregnancy. It should be noted that safe management of bipolar disorder during pregnancy also includes various other treatment modalities not included in this review. Psychotherapy, promotion of sleep hygiene, family education, substance abuse treatment, and electroconvulsive therapy, among others, may play important roles as well (Electroconvulsive therapy is discussed in Andrade C, Arumugham SS, Thirthalli J: Adverse Effects of Electroconvulsive Therapy, in this issue).

REFERENCES

1. Merikangas KR, Jin R, He JP, et al. Prevalence and correlates of bipolar spectrum disorder in the World Mental Health Survey Initiative. Arch Gen Psychiatry 2011; 68(3):241–51.
2. Miller C, Bauer MS. Excess mortality in bipolar disorders. Curr Psychiatry Rep 2014;16(11):499.
3. Angst F, Stassen HH, Clayton PJ, et al. Mortality of patients with mood disorders: follow-up over 34-38 years. J Affect Disord 2002;68(2–3):167–81.
4. Judd LL, Schettler PJ, Solomon DA, et al. Psychosocial disability and work role function compared across the long-term course of bipolar I, bipolar II, and unipolar major depressive disorders. J Affect Disord 2008;108(1–2):49–58.
5. Merikangas KR, Akiskal HS, Angst J, et al. Lifetime and 12-month prevalence of bipolar spectrum disorder in the national comorbidity survey replication. Arch Gen Psychiatry 2007;64:543–52.
6. Freeman MP, Smith KW, Freeman SA, et al. The impact of reproductive events on the course of bipolar disorder in women. J Clin Psychiatry 2002;63(4):284–7.
7. Di Florio A, Forty L, Gordon-Smith K, et al. Perinatal episodes across the mood disorder spectrum. JAMA Psychiatry 2013;70(2):168–75.
8. Viguera AC, Whitfield T, Baldessarini RJ, et al. Risk of recurrence in women with bipolar disorder during pregnancy: prospective study of mood stabilizer discontinuation. Am J Psychiatry 2007;164(12):1817–24.
9. Jones I. Bipolar disorder and childbirth: the importance of recognizing risk. Br J Psychiatry 2005;186:453–4.
10. Viguera AC, Tondo L, Koukopoulos AE, et al. Episodes of mood disorders in 2,252 pregnancies and postpartum periods. Am J Psychiatry 2011;168(11): 1179–85.
11. Boden R, Lundgren M, Brandt L, et al. Risks of adverse pregnancy and birth outcomes in women treated or not treated with mood stabilizers for bipolar disorder: population based cohort study. BMJ 2012;345:e7085.
12. Lee HC, Lin HC. Maternal bipolar disorder increased low birthweight and preterm births: a nationwide population-based study. J Affect Disord 2010;121(1–2):100–5.
13. Judd F, Komiti A, Sheehan P, et al. Adverse obstetric and neonatal outcomes in women with severe mental illness: to what extent can they be prevented? Schizophr Res 2014;157(1–3):305–9.

14. Nguyen TN, Faulkner D, Frayne JS, et al. Obstetric and neonatal outcomes of pregnant women with severe mental illness at a specialist antenatal clinic. Med J Aust 2013;199(3):S26–9.

15. Sit D, Rothschild A, Wisner K. A review of postpartum psychosis. J Womens Health 2011;15(4):352–68.

16. Centers for Disease Control and Prevention. Update on overall prevalence of major birth defects–Atlanta, Georgia, 1978-2005. MMWR Morb Mortal Wkly Rep 2008;57(1):1–5.

17. Hirschfeld R, Bowden C, Gitlin M, et al. Practice guideline for the treatment of patients with bipolar disorder. Focus 2003;1(1):64–110.

18. Bove EL, Hirsch JC, Ohye RG, et al. How I manage neonatal Ebstein's anomaly. Semin Thorac Cardiovasc Surg Pediatr Card Surg Annu 2009;63–5.

19. Cohen LS, Friedman JM, Jefferson JW, et al. A reevaluation of risk of in utero exposure to lithium. JAMA 1994;271(2):146–50.

20. Newport DJ, Viguera AC, Beach AJ, et al. Lithium placental passage and obstetrical outcome: implications for clinical management during late pregnancy. Am J Psychiatry 2005;162(11):2162–70.

21. McKnight RF, Adida M, Budge K, et al. Lithium toxicity profile: a systemic review and meta-analysis. Lancet 2012;379(9817):721–8.

22. Diav-Citrin O, Shechtman S, Tahover E, et al. Pregnancy outcome following in utero exposure to lithium: a prospective, comparative, observational study. Am J Psychiatry 2014;171(7):785–94.

23. Yacobi S, Ornoy A. Is lithium a real teratogen? What can we conclude from the prospective versus retrospective studies? A review. Isr J Psychiatry Relat Sci 2008;45(2):95–106.

24. Nguyen HTT, Sharma V, McIntyre R. Teratogenesis associated with antibipolar agents. Adv Ther 2009;26(3):281–94.

25. Wesseloo R, Kamperman AM, Munk-Olsen T, et al. Risk of postpartum relapse in bipolar disorder and postpartum psychosis: a systematic review and meta-analysis. Am J Psychiatry 2016;173(2):117–27.

26. Schou M. What happened later to the lithium babies? A follow-up study of children born without malformations. Acta Psychiatr Scand 1976;54(3):193–7.

27. Van der Lugt NM, Van de Maat JS, Van Kamp IL, et al. Fetal, neonatal and developmental outcomes of lithium-exposed pregnancies. Early Hum Dev 2012;88(6):375–8.

28. Bergink V, Kushner A. Lithium during pregnancy. Am J Psychiatry 2014;171(7):712–5.

29. Deligiannidis KM, Byatt N, Freeman MP. Pharmacotherapy for mood disorders in pregnancy: a review of pharmacokinetic changes and clinical recommendations for therapeutic drug monitoring. J Clin Psychopharmacol 2014;34(2):244–55.

30. Blake LD, Lucas DN, Aziz K, et al. Lithium toxicity and the parturient: case report and literature review. Int J Obstet Anesth 2008;17(2):164–9.

31. Viguera AC, Newport DJ, Ritchie J, et al. Lithium in breast milk and nursing infants: clinical implications. Am J Psychiatry 2007;164(2):342–5.

32. Bogen DL. Three cases of lithium exposure and exclusive breastfeeding. Arch Womens Ment Health 2012;15(1):69–72.

33. Howard LM, Megnin-Viggars O, Symington I, et al. Antenatal and postnatal mental health: summary of updated NICE guidance. BMJ 2014;349:g7394.

34. Hernandez-Diaz S, Smith CR, Shen A, et al. Comparative safety of antiepileptic drugs during pregnancy. Neurology 2012;78(21):1692–9.

35. Tomson T, Battino D, Bonizzoni E, et al. Dose-dependent risk of malformations with antiepileptic drugs: an analysis of data from the EURAP epilepsy and pregnancy registry. Lancet Neurol 2011;10(7):609–17.
36. Wyszynski DF, Nambisan M, Surve T, et al. Increased rate of major malformations in offspring exposed to valproate during pregnancy. Neurology 2005;64(6): 961–5.
37. Jentink J, Loane MA, Dolk H, et al. Valproic acid monotherapy in pregnancy and major congenital malformations. N Engl J Med 2010;362:2185–93.
38. Veiby G, Daltveit AK, Engelsen BA, et al. Fetal growth restriction and birth defects with newer and older antiepileptic drugs during pregnancy. J Neurol 2014;261(3): 579–88.
39. Ebbesen F, Joergensen A, Hoseth E, et al. Neonatal hypoglycaemia and withdrawal symptoms after exposure in utero to valproate. Arch Dis Child Fetal Neonatal Ed 2000;83(2):124–9.
40. Pearlstein T. Use of psychotropic medication during pregnancy and the post-partum period. Womens Health 2013;9(6):605–15.
41. Meador KJ, Baker GA, Browning N, et al. Fetal antiepileptic drug exposure and cognitive outcomes at age 6 years (NEAD study): a prospective observational study. Lancet Neurol 2013;12(3):244–52.
42. Morris JC, Meador KJ, Browning N, et al. Fetal antiepileptic drug exposure: adaptive and emotional/behavioral functioning at age 6 years. Epilepsy Behav 2013; 29(2):308–15.
43. Christensen J, Gronborg TK, Sorensen MJ, et al. Prenatal valproate exposure and risk of autism spectrum disorders and childhood autism. JAMA 2013;309(16): 1696–703.
44. Chaudron LH, Jefferson JW. Mood stabilizers during breastfeeding: a review. J Clin Psychiatry 2000;61(2):79–90.
45. Menon SJ. Psychotropic medication during pregnancy and lactation. Arch Gynecol Obstet 2008;277(1):1–13.
46. Cunnington MC, Weil JG, Messenheimer JS, et al. Final results from 18 years of the International Lamotrigine Pregnancy Registry. Neurology 2011;76(21): 1817–23.
47. Campbell E, Kennedy F, Russell A, et al. Malformation risks of antiepileptic drug monotherapies in pregnancy: updated results from the UK and Ireland Epilepsy and Pregnancy Registers. J Neurol Neurosurg Psychiatry 2014;85:1029–34.
48. Cummings C, Stewart M, Stevenson M, et al. Neurodevelopment of children exposed in utero to lamotrigine, sodium valproate and carbamazepine. Arch Dis Child 2011;96:643–7.
49. Bromley RL, Mawer GE, Briggs M, et al. The prevalence of neurodevelopmental disorders in children prenatally exposed to antiepileptic drugs. J Neurol Neurosurg Psychiatry 2013;84:637–43.
50. Clark CT, Klein AM, Perel JM, et al. Lamotrigine dosing for pregnant patients with bipolar disorder. Am J Psychiatry 2013;170(11):1240–7.
51. Reimers A, Helde G, Brodtkorb E. Ethinyl estradiol, not progestogens, reduces lamotrigine serum concentrations. Epilepsia 2005;46(9):1414–7.
52. Fotopoulou C, Kretz R, Bauer S, et al. Prospectively assessed changes in lamotrigine-concentration in women with epilepsy during pregnancy, lactation and the neonatal period. Epilepsy Res 2009;85(1):60–4.
53. Nordmo E, Aronsen L, Wasland K, et al. Severe apnea in an infant exposed to lamotrigine in breast milk. Ann Pharmacother 2009;43(11):1893–7.

54. Jentink J, Dolk H, Loane MA, et al. Intrauterine exposure to carbamazepine and specific congenital malformations: systemic review and case-control study. BMJ 2010;341:c6581.

55. Almgren M, Kallen B, Lavebratt C, et al. Population-based study of antiepileptic drug exposure in utero—influence on head circumference in newborns. Seizure 2009;18(10):672–5.

56. Cohen MJ, Meador KJ, Browning N, et al. Fetal antiepileptic drug exposure: motor, adaptive and emotional/behavioral functioning at age 3 years. Epilepsy Behav 2011;22(2):240–6.

57. Sabers A. Pharmacokinetic interactions between contraceptives and antiepileptic drugs. Seizure 2008;17(2):141–4.

58. Pennell PB, Gidal BE, Sabers A, et al. Pharmacology of antiepileptic drugs during pregnancy and lactation. Epilepsy Behav 2007;11(3):263–9.

59. Galbally M, Snellen M, Power J. Antipsychotic drugs in pregnancy: a review of their maternal and fetal effects. Ther Adv Drug Saf 2014;5(2):100–9.

60. Einarson A, Boskovic R. Use and safety of antipsychotic drugs during pregnancy. J Psychiatr Pract 2009;15:183–92.

61. Altshuler LL, Cohen L, Szuba MP, et al. Pharmacologic management of psychiatric illness during pregnancy: dilemmas and guidelines. Am J Psychiatry 1996; 153(5):592–606.

62. Newham JJ, Thomas SH, MacRitchie K, et al. Birth weight of infants after maternal exposure to typical and atypical antipsychotics: prospective comparison study. Br J Psychiatry 2008;192(5):333–7.

63. Lin HC, Chen IJ, Chen YH, et al. Maternal schizophrenia and pregnancy outcome: does the use of antipsychotics make a difference? Schizophr Res 2010;116(1):55–60.

64. Auerbach JG, Hans SL, Marcus J, et al. Maternal psychotropic medication and neonatal behavior. Neurotoxicol Teratol 1992;14(6):399–406.

65. FDA Drug Safety Communication: Antipsychotic drug labels updated on use during pregnancy and risk of abnormal muscle movements and withdrawal symptoms in newborns. FDA; 2011. Available at: http://www.fda.gov/Drugs/DrugSafety/ucm243903.htm.

66. Kieviet N, Dolman KM, Honig A. The use of psychotropic medication during pregnancy: how about the newborn? Neuropsychiatr Dis Treat 2013;9:1257–66.

67. Slone D, Siskind V, Heinonen O, et al. Antenatal exposure to the phenothiazines in relation to congenital malformations, perinatal mortality rate, birth weight, and intelligence quotient score. Am J Obstet Gynecol 1977;128:486–8.

68. Patton SW, Misri S, Corral MR, et al. Antipsychotic medication during pregnancy and lactation in women with schizophrenia: evaluating the risk. Can J Psychiatry 2002;47(10):959–65.

69. McKenna K, Koren G, Tetelbaum M, et al. Pregnancy outcome of women using atypical antipsychotic drugs: a prospective comparative study. J Clin Psychiatry 2005;66(4):444–9.

70. Habermann F, Fritzsche J, Fuhlbruck F, et al. Atypical antipsychotic drugs and pregnancy outcome: a prospective, cohort study. J Clin Psychopharmacol 2013;33(4):453–62.

71. Kulkarni J, Worsley R, Gilbert H, et al. A prospective cohort study of antipsychotic medications in pregnancy: the first 147 pregnancies and 100 one year old babies. PLoS One 2014;9(5):e94788.

72. Sadowski A, Todorow M, Brojeni PY, et al. Pregnancy outcomes following maternal exposure to second-generation antipsychotics given with other psychotropic drugs: a cohort study. BMJ Open 2013;3(7):e003062.
73. Cohen LS, Viguera AC, McInerney KA, et al. Reproductive safety of second-generation antipsychotics: current data from the Massachusetts General Hospital National Pregnancy Registry for atypical antipsychotics. Am J Psychiatry 2016; 173(3):263–70.
74. Babu GN, Desai G, Tippeswamy H, et al. Birth weight and use of olanzapine in pregnancy: a prospective comparative study. J Clin Psychopharmacol 2010;30:331–2.
75. Newport DJ, Calamaras MR, DeVane CL, et al. Atypical antipsychotic administration during late pregnancy: placental passage and obstetrical outcomes. Am J Psychiatry 2007;164:1214–20.
76. Newcomer JW. Antipsychotic medications: metabolic and cardiovascular risk. J Clin Psychiatry 2007;68(Suppl 4):8–13.
77. Hironaka M, Kotani S, Sumigama H, et al. Maternal mental disorders and pregnancy outcomes: a clinical study in a Japanese population. J Obstet Gynaecol Res 2011;37(10):1283–9.
78. Boden R, Lundgren M, Brandt L, et al. Antipsychotics during pregnancy: relation to fetal and maternal metabolic effects. Arch Gen Psychiatry 2012;69(7):715–21.
79. Reis M, Bengt K. Maternal use of antipsychotics in early pregnancy and delivery outcome. J Clin Psychopharmacol 2008;28(3):279–88.
80. Stiegler A, Schaletzky R, Walter G, et al. Olanzapine treatment during pregnancy and breastfeeding: a chance for women with psychotic illness? Psychopharmacology 2014;231(15):3067–9.
81. Aichhorn W, Stuppaeck C, Whitworth AB. Risperidone and breast-feeding. J Psychopharmacol 2005;19(2):211–3.
82. Lee A, Giesbrecht E, Dunn E, et al. Excretion of quetiapine in breast milk. Am J Psychiatry 2004;161(9):1715–6.
83. Brunner E, Falk DM, Jones M, et al. Olanzapine in pregnancy and breastfeeding: a review of data from global safety surveillance. BMC Pharmacol Toxicol 2013;14:38.
84. Wittkowski A, McGrath LK, Peters S. Exploring psychosis and bipolar disorder in women: a critical review of the qualitative literature. BMC Psychiatry 2014;14:281.
85. Finer LB, Zolna MR. Declines in unintended pregnancy in the United States, 2008-2011. N Engl J Med 2016;374(9):843–52.
86. Marengo E, Martino DJ, Igoa A, et al. Unplanned pregnancies and reproductive health among women with bipolar disorder. J Affect Disord 2015;178:201–5.

Adverse Effects of Second-Generation Antipsychotics as Adjuncts to Antidepressants
Are the Risks Worth the Benefits?

Michael E. Thase, MD

KEYWORDS

- Adverse effects • Second-generation antipsychotics • Adjunctive therapy • Risks
- Benefits

KEY POINTS

- Using attrition due to adverse effects as the indicator of harm, the number needed to harm in short-term clinical trials ranges from 8 to 20 (ie, 5% to 12% risk differences in attrition).
- There are meaningful differences in the incidence of specific adverse effects, with akathisia more common with aripiprazole, sedation more common with quetiapine extended release, and weight gain more common with olanzapine.
- Duration of therapy is an important determinant of longer-term risks, and careful monitoring of weight and related metabolic parameters is indicated during continuation pharmacotherapy; cases of tardive dyskinesia have been observed within the first year of continued adjunctive second-generation antipsychotics (SGA) therapy.
- Although the benefits of adjunctive therapy with SGAs can be considerable, treatment with these adjuncts appears most indicated for depressed patients who are unlikely to respond to alternate strategies and for whom the rapidity of benefit (eg, inpatient status, marked impairment, or worsening symptom severity) justifies the several risks.

Financial Disclosure: During the last 3 years, Dr M.E. Thase reports earning fees as a consultant to Alkermes, Allergan, AstraZeneca, Avenir, Aventis, Bristol-Myers Squibb, Cerecor, Eli Lilly & Co, Forest Laboratories, Gerson Lehman Group, GlaxoSmithKline, Guidepoint Global, Janssen (Johnson & Johnson), H. Lundbeck A/S, MedAvante, Inc, Merck, Naurex, Neuronetics Inc, Novartis, Otsuka, Nestle (PamLab), Pfizer, Roche Inc, Shire US Inc, Sunovion, and Takeda. During the same timeframe, he has received research grants from Agency for Healthcare Research and Quality, Alkermes, AstraZeneca, Assurex, Avenir, Eli Lilly & Co, Forest Pharmaceuticals, GlaxoSmithKline, Janssen (Johnson & Johnson), the National Institute of Mental Health, Otsuka Pharmaceuticals, Pharmaneuroboost, Roche, and Takeda. Dr M.E. Thase's spouse is an employee of Peloton Advantage, which does business with several pharmaceutical companies.
Mood and Anxiety Treatment and Research Program, Perelman School of Medicine, University of Pennsylvania, 3535 Market Street, Suite 670, Philadelphia, PA 19104-3309, USA
E-mail address: thase@mail.med.upenn.edu

Psychiatr Clin N Am 39 (2016) 477–486
http://dx.doi.org/10.1016/j.psc.2016.04.008
0193-953X/16/$ – see front matter

INTRODUCTION

Major depressive disorder (MDD) is one of the world's great public health problems and, until recently, development of safe and effective novel antidepressant medications was one of the top priorities of the pharmaceutical industry. These efforts have led to development of several newer classes of medications that have largely supplanted older standards, including "classic" drugs such as the tricyclic antidepressants (TCAs) and monoamine oxidase inhibitors (MAOIs), as the antidepressants of first choice throughout most of the economically developed world. However, the advantages of the newer medications over the TCAs and MAOIs were in areas such as ease of use, tolerability, and safety in overdose, not efficacy. The newer antidepressants are, in fact, either no more effective or slightly less so than the older standards. As the use of antidepressants has skyrocketed since the introduction of fluoxetine in late 1987 ushered in the modern era of antidepressant therapy, so too has the problem of antidepressant nonresponse. This problem is mammoth in scope, because as many as 10% of the adult US population now take antidepressants and only about one-half of the depressed patients who begin pharmacotherapy will experience at least a 50% reduction in symptom intensity (ie, a minimal definition of response) after 6 to 8 weeks of therapy with an adequate dose of medication.[1] There is evidence that the problem of antidepressant nonresponse grows progressively as the number of failed treatment trials mounts. For example, about 60% of those who continue on for a second course of treatment will not respond, and after 4 trials, about 30% of patients will still be depressed.[1] Patients who have not responded to 2 sequential, adequate courses of antidepressant medication are considered by some experts and regulatory guidelines alike to meet the minimum definition of treatment-resistant depression (TRD).[2] In one large-scale study known as Sequenced Treatments Alternatives to Relieve Depression (STAR*D),[1] for example, patients who had not responded to 2 trials of newer-generation antidepressants had less than a 20% chance of remission with subsequent monotherapy trials with 2 of the old favorites, the TCA nortriptyline and the MAOI tranylcypromine. Because patients with TRD account for a disproportionately large share of the burden/disability associated with MDD,[3] developing safe and effective strategies for them represents one of the most important topics in psychiatric therapeutics. It is within this context that adjunctive therapy with second-generation antipsychotics (SGA) has emerged as one of the leading options for patients with TRD. This article considers the benefits of adjunctive SGA therapy as well as the risks.

OVERVIEW OF TREATMENT-RESISTANT DEPRESSION

Although clinicians often think about TRD as a categorical entity (ie, either you meet the criteria or you do not), patients' histories and patterns of response and nonresponse vary dramatically across several dimensions. At the most superficial level, it seems unlikely that someone who has not responded to two 6-week courses of selective serotonin reuptake inhibitor (SSRI) therapy at minimum doses has the same prognosis as someone who has not responded to 12 months of continuous therapy with 4 different classes of medication. Conversely, although clinicians often consider electroconvulsive therapy (ECT) to be the sine qua non of biological therapies for severe depression, it is unlikely that this venerable treatment, which is more intensive, invasive, and costly than most other strategies, would be considered the most appropriate option for the first patient described above, but many would agree that it is a reasonable next step for the second patient. Similar decisions apply to the use of older medications, such as the TCAs, MAOIs, and lithium salts, at earlier time points. Thus, an algorithmic or hierarchical perspective is one of the relevant dimensions necessary to better describe a patient who is said to have TRD. The staging system for TRD proposed in the mid-1990s by Thase and Rush,[4] for example, was explicitly hierarchical and extended from nonresponse to one adequate course of a first-line medication (eg, an SSRI or, at the time, TCA) and extended through trials of alternate newer and older medications, with nonresponse to ECT representing the most advanced or resistant level (ie, stage V TRD).

In retrospect, the staging system proposed by Thase and Rush,[4] which was drawn from the schema used by oncologists to stage malignancies, conflated temporal progression or chronicity of depressive illness with treatment history. Treatment resistance is actually not a diagnosis, but rather a description of one aspect of the patients' longitudinal illness course. Thus, it is probably more accurate to refer to levels of treatment resistance rather than actual stages. Nevertheless, it is true that patients with more advanced levels of treatment resistance are less responsive to standard therapies and may well require treatments that have targets other than serotonin and/or norepinephrine transporters. As noted above, in 2016, this issue is most pertinent for patients who have not responded to at least 2 trials of SSRIs, serotonin norepinephrine reuptake inhibitors (SNRIs), or other "first-line" antidepressants. Within such a contemporary context, the clinical decision of greatest import for such a patient with a less advanced form of TRD pertains to what to do next: should I switch to another antidepressant, should I combine 2 different antidepressants, or should I add an adjunct?

STRATEGIES OF TREATMENT-RESISTANT DEPRESSION: SWITCHING VERSUS ADDING

Before starting a new treatment for a patient with TRD, it is important to review the accuracy of the diagnosis, ensure that the patient has been adherent to the current treatment and has not been surreptitiously using large amounts of alcohol or drugs, and confirm that the past trials have been adequate in terms of both duration and dose. Although many of the newer antidepressants do not have crisply delineated dose-response relationships, it is generally a good idea to optimize the index course of therapy by titrating the dose up to the maximum approved dose, if tolerability permits. When the adequacy of the current course of therapy is in doubt, a conservative yet very reasonable strategy is to extend the treatment trial by 2 more weeks to see if the response status has become clearer.

When a course of antidepressant therapy has been optimized but is still not effective, the tolerability of the index antidepressant is one of the keys to deciding what to do next. If tolerability is marginal or worse, the decision is easy: switch to a dissimilar antidepressant. When the index therapy is well tolerated and there has been some improvement, many psychiatrists will now opt for adding an adjunct rather than switching. Using an adjunct in this clinical context not only conveys the advantage of a building on an established therapy but also avoids any worsening that might result from tapering and cross-titration.[2] Five "add-on" strategies were evaluated in STAR*D, including 3 medications that are not classified as antidepressants (buspirone, lithium, and the T_3 form of thyroid hormone) and 2 antidepressants (bupropion and mirtazapine).[1] Many consider the use of 2 antidepressants together a special case (ie, combination therapy) and reserve the term adjunctive therapy for medications that are not approved antidepressants, although this distinction is largely semantic.

The deceptively simple question "is it better to switch or use an adjunct?" is not so easily answered. Even the massive STAR*D study, which planned comparison of adjunctive and switching strategies across all 3 randomized levels, did not point to clear answers, although, across levels, patients who received adjunctive therapies were more likely to remit than those who were switched to another course of antidepressant monotherapy.[1] However, because the study used a special form of randomization that preserved patient/clinician choice of strategies whenever possible, those who opted for adjunctive strategies reported lower levels of depressive symptoms and fewer adverse effects with the index medication, which are indicators of being easier to treat.[1] Nevertheless, the STAR*D clinicians were able to implement adjunctive strategies faster than they were able to orchestrate switches, and ease of implementation is an important advantage when efficacy/effectiveness appears to be comparable.

SECOND-GENERATION ANTIPSYCHOTICS: THE NEW STANDARD FOR ADJUNCTIVE THERAPY FOR TREATMENT-RESISTANT DEPRESSION?

Adding an antipsychotic medication to an antidepressant is actually one of the oldest adjunctive therapies, and first-generation antipsychotics were commonly used in combination with TCAs and MAOIs in the 1960s and 1970s. However, this practice largely fell out of favor by the 1980s, in part because the risk of tardive dyskinesia associated with therapy with antipsychotic medications was thought to be particularly high for people with mood disorders. It is also true that other, potentially safer adjunctive strategies, including added thyroid hormone or lithium salts, were introduced in the 1980s and, by the early 1990s, the once taboo practice of combining antidepressants experienced a renaissance as clinicians began to use SSRIs in combination with TCAs or bupropion.[2]

The perception that it was inappropriate to use antipsychotic medications to treat patients with nonpsychotic depressive disorders began to change shortly after the introduction of the first members of a newer or so-called second generation of antipsychotics.[5] The small early study of Shelton and colleagues,[6] which examined fluoxetine and olanzapine, singly and in combination, in patients who had not responded to antidepressants alone was particularly influential. Across the next 10+ years, the adjunctive use of SGAs for antidepressant nonresponders skyrocketed,[7] and, although exact data are lacking, it appears that the SGAs are now the most widely used form of adjunctive therapy for antidepressant nonresponders. As reviewed by Nelson and Papakostas,[8] there are multiple positive placebo-controlled studies for 4 SGAs, including the 3 drugs that have been approved by the US Food and Drug Administration (FDA) for a specific indication (aripiprazole, quetiapine, and olanzapine), and a fourth (risperidone) that was not formally submitted for review by the FDA for this indication. Recently, a fifth SGA (brexpiprazole) was approved by the FDA on the basis of 2 positive studies.[9,10] In practice, all 4 of these medications show relatively rapid clinical benefits, which, if they are going to occur, almost invariably are observed within 1 to 2 weeks.[2] Moreover, the adjunctive efficacy of these drugs is typically observed at doses that are only one-fourth to one/half those used to treat acute schizophrenia or mania.[2] Thus, in this clinical context, it would appear that the antidepressant effects of these medications are not directly tied to their antipsychotic effects. With so many members of the SGA class showing such positive findings, including drugs as dissimilar as risperidone and quetiapine or olanzapine and aripiprazole, it is very likely that antidepressant effects are common across the whole class. Consistent with this speculation, a positive study has been recently reported for ziprasidone,[11] and a series of studies of cariprazine are nearing completion.[12]

TOLERABILITY OF ADJUNCTIVE SECOND-GENERATION ANTIPSYCHOTICS THERAPY
Short-Term Studies

Discontinuation due to adverse events
Although the use of intent-to-treat analyses of efficacy takes the impact of premature attrition from therapy into account, poor tolerability is not the only reason that patients discontinue treatment. Thus, a better global measure of tolerability is the proportion of patients who discontinue because of intolerable adverse effects. For randomized controlled trials (RCTs) that include a placebo control group, a simple risk difference (discontinuation rate on drug minus that on placebo) is a useful indicator of tolerability, with statistical significance. In one meta-analysis,[8] which included data from 16 placebo-controlled studies of adjunctive SGA therapy, 9.1% of the patients receiving an adjunctive SGA discontinued the SGA because of intolerable adverse effects, compared with 2.3% of the patients receiving a placebo adjunct, resulting in a risk difference of 6.8%. This hazard corresponds to number needed to harm (NNH) of 14. Thus, adjunctive SGA therapy conveys a risk of discontinuation of treatment that is somewhat higher than that typically observed in studies of first-line pharmacotherapies (eg, NNH values of 15–25),[13] but comparable to the discontinuation rates observed for the TCA and MAOI arms in STAR*D.[1]

More recently, Zhou and colleagues[14] conducted a systematic review and network meta-analysis of a larger pool of studies of adjunctive therapy for MDD; tolerability analyses included data from 39 studies, including 17 RCTs of adjunctive SGAs. They concluded that attrition (drug vs placebo differences) due to intolerable adverse effects were roughly comparable for aripiprazole, olanzapine, quetiapine, and risperidone. In terms of effect sizes, Zhou and colleagues computed odds ratios (drug relative to placebo) that ranged from 2.5 (aripiprazole and risperidone) to 3.4 (olanzapine) and 3.9 (quetiapine). If one assumes an attrition rate of 2% to 3% for ongoing antidepressant therapy plus placebo,[8] then the estimated risk differences for adjunctive SGA therapy would range from about 5% to 9%, which essentially replicates the conclusion of Nelson and Papakostas' finding using a different statistical method.

One important characteristic of the network meta-analytic method used by Zhou and colleagues[14] is the ability to make indirect comparisons of the tolerability of adjunctive SGA therapy with other widely used adjunctive strategies. Although one must be cautious in interpreting such indirect comparison because of the possibility of bias, the results do suggest that the tolerability of adjunctive SGA therapy is somewhat worse than that of other widely used strategies, including adjunctive thyroid hormone, lithium salts, psychostimulants, and bupropion. However, the only large-scale study to directly compare adjunctive strategies in patients with TRD[15] found no significant differences in tolerability between adjunctive quetiapine extended release (300 mg/d; n = 231) or lithium therapy (0.6–1.2 mEq/L; n = 229). A second large-scale study that compares adjunctive aripiprazole versus adjunctive bupropion has recently been completed, and preliminary results should be available in late 2016.[16]

Akathisia
Although there does not appear to be a meaningful difference in the overall hazard of dropping out of therapy with SGAs, there are important differences in the specific adverse effects that emerge during adjunctive therapy. In short, akathisia and

restlessness are the most common problematic adverse effects associated with adjunctive therapy with aripiprazole and brexpiprazole; sedation is the most common problematic adverse effect associated with adjunctive quetiapine therapy, and increased appetite and weight gain are the most problematic adverse effects associated with adjunctive therapy with olanzapine.[17–19] If NNH values are computed on the incidence of adverse effects, rather than attrition due to intolerable adverse effects, a much harsher view of tolerability is revealed.[13,16] For example, because about one-half of patients treated with quetiapine will report some degree of sedation or daytime sleepiness during the first week of therapy (compared with <10% on placebo), an NNH value of 3 can be estimated. Likewise, a pooled rate of about 33% for akathisia and restlessness on adjunctive aripiprazole, compared with less than 5% on placebo, would result in an NNH estimate of 4. Clearly, the risks of adjunctive SGA therapy are heavily dependent on the definition of harm.

Weight gain

As most of the SGAs convey some risk of weight gain, and weight gain in short-term trials is a valuable indicator of subsequent risk of a range of metabolic difficulties (ie, obesity, dyslipidemia, and glucose intolerance), the comparative risks of weight gain during adjunctive SGA therapy is an important determinant of which medication to pick.[17,18] Clinicians can take some comfort in the fact that weight can be measured so accurately and inexpensively. Spielmans and colleagues[17] included weight change in their systematic review and meta-analysis. For olanzapine, which was only systematically studied in combination with fluoxetine (5 studies), an average weight gain of 4.2 kg was observed in controlled studies lasting up to 10 weeks. Mean weight gain in the 3 RCTs of adjunctive aripiprazole was much lower (1.1 kg). However, these studies were only 6 weeks in duration. In the 3 controlled studies of adjunctive quetiapine, which permitted a larger number of antidepressants, mean weight gain was 0.9 kg across up to 8 weeks of double-blind therapy. Weight gain across 4 to 6 weeks of double-blind adjunctive risperidone therapy was 1.3 kg. Although not included in this meta-analysis,[17] the 2 RCTs of brexpiprazole (1–3 mg/d) demonstrated a comparable amount of about 1.5-kg weight gain across 6 weeks of double-blind therapy.[9,10] Across individuals treated with adjunctive SGAs, the risk of weight gain is not normally distributed, and a relatively low mean weight gain of about 1 kg actually reflects a large (eg, 7%) weight gain for 5% to 10% of patients.

Longer-Term Studies

There are only a few longer-term, controlled studies of adjunctive SGA therapy in patients with MDD. To date, there are only 2 placebo-controlled studies of continuation phase therapy across 6 months of follow-up: one evaluating risperidone in combination with citalopram[20] and the other evaluating the combination of fixed doses of olanzapine and fluoxetine.[21]

The first study evaluated adjunctive risperidone therapy (0.5–2.0 mg/d) in 386 MDD patients who did not respond to a prospective trial of up to 6 weeks of citalopram monotherapy (20–60 mg/d).[20] A total of 243 patients responded to 4 to 6 weeks of adjunctive therapy and enrolled in the double-blind, placebo-controlled discontinuation trial. Of these patients, attrition due to adverse effects during continuation phase therapy was 4.1% on adjunctive risperidone therapy compared with 2.5% for the group receiving adjunctive placebo. The mean weight change during the double-blind phase was 1.3 (3.8) kg for the group receiving active risperidone and −0.5 (2.9) kg for the group receiving adjunctive placebo during the continuation phase. A total of 8.3% of the patients receiving active risperidone and citalopram therapy report significant weight gain (as defined by a 7% increase in weight) over and above the number who gained weight during open-label therapy, compared with only 2.6% of the patients receiving citalopram and a placebo adjunct. If this difference is used to compute NNH for continuation therapy, one patient would be harmed by weight gain for every 20 patients who responded to adjunctive therapy with risperidone. Other significant changes noted during the continuation phase pertaining to patient safety involved plasma prolactin and reports of galactorrhea (2.5% vs 0%); both differences were significantly higher in the group receiving active risperidone. There were no cases of tardive dyskinesia observed during the 6 months of double-blind therapy. Although the risks associated with longer-term adjunctive risperidone therapy were modest, it must be noted that the benefit-risk ratio observed in this study is not favorable because the drug versus placebo difference in relapse prevention was not statistically significant across the 6 months of double-blind therapy. Although secondary analyses did suggest better prophylaxis in subsets of risperidone-treated patients, this failed trial was instrumental in the manufacturer's decision not to pursue a formal indication for adjunctive treatment of MDD.

The second study[21] enrolled 892 MDD patients with a history of nonresponse to at least 2 adequate courses of antidepressant monotherapy. A total of 655 patients showed some degree of response to 6 weeks of open-label therapy with olanzapine-fluoxetine combination (OFC) and entered a 12-week stabilization phase, of which 444 patients met response criteria and accepted randomization to either ongoing OFC (n = 221) or fluoxetine monotherapy (n = 223). During the 6-month double-blind continuation phase, 19 patients (8.6%) withdrew from the OFC arm because of intolerable adverse effects, as compared with 10 patients (4.5%) receiving fluoxetine monotherapy (NNH = 25). Because preventive therapy with OFC reduced the risk of relapse by 50% (32% to 16%; NNT = 7), the benefit-to-risk ratio was judged to be favorable. However, clinically significant weight gain during the 6 additional months of therapy was problematic for the OFC group, with 11.8% of patients experiencing a 7% weight gain as compared with 2.3% of the group that was switched to fluoxetine monotherapy (NNH = 10). Although only 5% of the group taking OFC experienced a clinically significant ($\geq$7%) weight loss during continuation phase therapy, 15.3% of the group switched to fluoxetine monotherapy and was able to lose a clinically significant amount of weight. If these mutually exclusive hazards are added together as a composite risk, the NNH for weight-related issues during continuation OFC therapy is 5. Perhaps most importantly, the risk of significant weight gain was 50% for the patients who completed all 3 phases or 9 months of therapy with OFC, corresponding to an NNH of 2. The magnitude of this risk suggests that olanzapine, whether in combination with fluoxetine or another SSRI or SNRI, ordinarily should not be one of the first SGA options considered, and when it is used, stringent monitoring of weight and metabolic parameters (see later discussion) is indicated.

RECOMMENDATIONS TO MINIMIZE RISK

The best way to minimize risk is to limit prescription of SGAs to only those patients who have relatively severe symptoms and/or there is an urgent need for clinical benefit. When the potential for benefit is judged on clinical grounds to offset the risks, treatment should be continued beyond 6 weeks only when there has been an unequivocal response. At the outset of treatment, weight should be recorded and, if clinically indicated, a baseline battery that includes a fasting plasma glucose level and a lipid panel should be obtained.[18] As the optimal duration of therapy has not been established, it is reasonable to consider tapering down the adjunctive medications within a few months of therapy. If symptomatic worsening dictates continuing adjunctive SGA therapy longer than a few months, the absence of neurologic signs of TD should be documented and, if baseline laboratory parameters were not obtained at the outset of therapy, a baseline should be established and periodically repeated if the duration of therapy extends beyond 6 months.

It is generally a good idea to establish an agreed on "maximum acceptable weight gain" and monitor this at each visit; for many, a 2- to 5-kg weight gain will be considered a realistic maximum. Trends in weight gain over time need to be recognized and addressed vigorously. Weight gain more than 2 kg per month is worrisome and requires a level of intervention; reducing dietary intake and increasing caloric expenditure by a net 500 Kcal per day is difficult for most to implement. Should the maximal weight gain value be reached, a change in treatment is in order. Although sometimes this can be accomplished by switching within the SGA class (eg, from quetiapine to aripiprazole or from aripiprazole to ziprasidone or lurasidone), often it is necessary to switch to a different strategy.

Given the deleterious prognosis of TD, in most cases the SGA should be stopped at the first sign of involuntary movements. Although clinical experience is limited during longer-term adjunctive therapy, there is reason to be optimistic that dyskinesias will resolve if the offending medication is stopped.[22]

SUMMARY

Adjunctive therapy with SGAs is now one the most widely used strategies for patients with TRD. From the perspective of evidence-based medicine, there is no better proven strategy for patients who have not responded to several courses of therapy with SSRIs, SNRIs, or other newer-generation antidepressants; there are 2 or more positive, placebo-controlled studies for aripiprazole, brexpiprazole, olanzapine, risperidone, and quetiapine. Beyond reproducibility of effect, there is rapidity of action: when effective, these medications usually produce meaningful symptom relief within 2 weeks.

The considerable potential benefits of the SGAs must be balanced against their cost and risks. Although risperidone, quetiapine, and aripiprazole are now available in generic formulations, the cost of generic SGAs is still considerably greater than the alternatives (eg, lithium, thyroid, or antidepressant combinations). Acquisition costs are of course amplified by the costs associated with monitoring for metabolic complications and/or those resulting from the need to treat dyslipidemia or obesity. Fortunately, treatment-emergent cases of diabetes mellitus or tardive dyskinesia are uncommon occurrences during adjunctive therapy with SGAs; nevertheless, these treatments are associated with significant medical morbidity that must be prevented whenever possible. As a result of these several concerns, although adjunctive therapy with an SGA should be thought of as one of the gold standards for treating antidepressant nonresponders, this should usually be used only when symptom severity or the urgency for rapid benefit is sufficient to justify the costs and potential risks.

REFERENCES

1. Rush AJ, Trivedi MH, Wisniewski SR, et al. Acute and longer-term outcomes in depressed outpatients requiring one or several treatment steps: a STAR*D report. Am J Psychiatry 1905;2006:163.
2. Connolly KR, Thase ME. If at first you don't succeed: a review of the evidence for antidepressant augmentation, combination and switching strategies. Drugs 2011;71:43–64.

3. Crown WH, Finkelstein S, Berndt ER, et al. The impact of treatment-resistant depression on health care utilization and costs. J Clin Psychiatry 2002;63:963–71.

4. Thase ME, Rush AJ. When at first you don't succeed: sequential strategies for antidepressant nonresponders. J Clin Psychiatry 1997;58(Suppl 13):23–9.

5. Thase ME. What role do atypical antipsychotic drugs have in treatment-resistant depression? J Clin Psychiatry 2002;63:95–103.

6. Shelton RC, Tollefson GD, Tohen M, et al. A novel augmentation strategy for treating resistant major depression. Am J Psychiatry 2001;158:131–4.

7. Gerhard T, Akincigil A, Correll CU, et al. National trends in second-generation antipsychotic augmentation for nonpsychotic depression. J Clin Psychiatry 2014;75:490–7.

8. Nelson JC, Papakostas GI. Atypical antipsychotic augmentation in major depressive disorder: a meta-analysis of placebo-controlled randomized trials. Am J Psychiatry 2009;166:980–91.

9. Thase ME, Youakim JM, Skuban A, et al. Adjunctive brexpiprazole 1 and 3 mg for patients with major depressive disorder following inadequate response to antidepressants: a phase 3, randomized, double-blind study. J Clin Psychiatry 2015;76:1232–40.

10. Thase ME, Youakim JM, Skuban A, et al. Efficacy and safety of adjunctive brexpiprazole 2 mg in major depressive disorder: a phase 3, randomized, placebo-controlled study in patients with inadequate response to antidepressants. J Clin Psychiatry 2015;76:1224–31.

11. Papakostas GI, Fava M, Baer L, et al. Ziprasidone augmentation of escitalopram for major depressive disorder: efficacy results from a randomized, double-blind, placebo-controlled study. Am J Psychiatry 2015;172:1251–8.

12. McCormack PL. Cariprazine: first global approval. Drugs 2015;75:2035–43.

13. Gao K, Kemp DE, Fein E, et al. Number needed to treat to harm for discontinuation due to adverse events in the treatment of bipolar depression, major depressive disorder, and generalized anxiety disorder with atypical antipsychotics. J Clin Psychiatry 2011;72(8):1063–71.

14. Zhou X, Keitner GI, Qin B, et al. Atypical antipsychotic augmentation for treatment-resistant depression: a systematic review and network meta-analysis. Int J Neuropsychopharmacol 2015;18(11):pyv060.

15. Bauer M, Dell'Osso L, Kasper S, et al. Extended-release quetiapine fumarate (quetiapine XR) monotherapy and quetiapine XR or lithium as add-on to antidepressants in patients with treatment-resistant major depressive disorder. J Affect Disord 2013;151:209–19.

16. Mohamed S, Johnson GR, Vertrees JE, et al. The VA augmentation and switching treatments for improving depression outcomes (VAST-D) study: rationale and design considerations. Psychiatry Res 2015;229:760–70.

17. Spielmans GI, Berman MI, Linardatos E, et al. Adjunctive atypical antipsychotic treatment for major depressive disorder: a meta-analysis of depression, quality of life and safety outcomes. PLoS Med 2013;10:e1001403.

18. DeBattista C, DeBattista K. Safety considerations of the use of second generation antipsychotics in the treatment of major depression: extrapyramidal and metabolic side effects [review]. Curr Drug Saf 2010;5(3):263–6.

19. Citrome L. Adjunctive aripiprazole, olanzapine, or quetiapine for major depressive disorder: an analysis of number needed to treat, number needed to harm, and likelihood to be helped or harmed. Postgrad Med 2010;122:39–48.

20. Rapaport MH, Gharabawi GM, Canuso CM, et al. Effects of risperidone augmentation in patients with treatment-resistant depression: results of open-label

treatment followed by double-blind continuation. Neuropsychopharmacology 2006;31:2505–13.

21. Brunner E, Tohen M, Osuntokun O, et al. Efficacy and safety of olanzapine/fluoxetine combination vs fluoxetine monotherapy following successful combination therapy of treatment-resistant major depressive disorder. Neuropsychopharmacology 2014; 39:2549–59.

22. Berman RM, Thase ME, Trivedi MH, et al. Long-term safety and tolerability of open-label aripiprazole augmentation of antidepressant therapy in major depressive disorder. Neuropsychiatr Dis Treat 2011;7:303–12.

Adverse Effects of Psychotropic Medications on Sleep

Karl Doghramji, MD[a],*, William C. Jangro, DO[b]

KEYWORDS

- Antidepressant • Antipsychotic • Insomnia • Sedation • Adverse effects • Sleep
- Somnolence

KEY POINTS

- Psychotropic medications have a broad range of mechanisms of action, which are presumed to be involved in their sleep-related adverse effects.
- Insomnia and daytime somnolence are common adverse effects of these medications.
- These effects can be beneficial or detrimental depending on the particular symptoms of the patient's psychiatric disorder.
- Being aware of an agent's most likely adverse effects on sleep can aid the prescriber in choosing an agent that is more likely to improve the sleep component of a patient's psychiatric disorder.

ANTIDEPRESSANTS

People suffering from depressive disorders typically complain of difficulty falling asleep, frequent awakenings, early morning wakening, and non-refreshing sleep. Polysomnographic studies of depressed persons have confirmed these findings and show reduced rapid eye movement (REM) latency, increased REMs, increased total time in REM sleep, reduced slow wave sleep (SWS), and frequent awakenings throughout the night.[1] Antidepressants are widely prescribed for mood and anxiety disorders. According to the National Health and Nutrition Examination Survey, 11% of Americans over the age of 12 are taking an antidepressant medication.[2] Most of

Dr K. Doghramji owns stock in Merck and is a consultant for Merck, Inspire, Jazz, Xenoport, Teva, Pfizer, and Pernix. Dr W. C. Jangro has nothing to disclose.

[a] Fellowship in Sleep Medicine, Department of Psychiatry and Human Behavior, Jefferson Sleep Disorders Center, Sidney Kimmel Medical College, Thomas Jefferson University, Walnut Towers, 5th Floor, 211 South 9th Street, Philadelphia, PA 19107, USA; [b] Adult Residency Training Program, Department of Psychiatry and Human Behavior, Sidney Kimmel Medical College, Thomas Jefferson University, 833 Chestnut Street, Suite 210, Philadelphia, PA 19107, USA
* Corresponding author.
E-mail address: karl.doghramji@jefferson.edu

Psychiatr Clin N Am 39 (2016) 487–502
http://dx.doi.org/10.1016/j.psc.2016.04.009
0193-953X/16/$ – see front matter © 2016 Elsevier Inc. All rights reserved.

psych.theclinics.com

488 Doghramji & Jangro

Abbreviations	
5-HT	5-Hydroxytryptamine
ADHD	Attention-deficit/hyperactivity disorder
H1	Histamine 1 receptor
MAOI	Monoamine oxidase inhibitor
MDD	Major depressive disorder
NNTH	Numbers needed to treat to harm
PLM	Periodic limb movement
PSG	Polysomnogram
PSQI	Pittsburgh Sleep Quality Index
REM	Rapid eye movement
RLS	Restless legs syndrome
SNRI	Serotonin-norepinephrine reuptake inhibitor
SOL	Sleep onset latency
SRED	Sleep-related eating disorders
SSRI	Selective serotonin reuptake inhibitor
SWS	Slow wave sleep
TCA	Tricyclic antidepressant
TST	Total sleep time
VLPO	Ventrolateral preoptic nucleus
WASO	Wakefulness after sleep onset

these antidepressant medications are thought to exert their effects through modulation of various monoamines as well as interactions with receptors such as histamine and muscarinic cholinergic receptors. Through these interactions, antidepressants can have a significant impact on sleep physiology. The central processes governing sleep and wakefulness are dependent on the complex interaction of these various neurotransmitter systems.[3,4] The ascending arousal system, which traverses from the brainstem regions to the cerebral cortex, consists of noradrenergic neurons of the ventrolateral medulla and locus coeruleus, cholinergic neurons in the pedunculopontine and laterodorsal tegmental nuclei, serotonergic neurons in the dorsal raphe nucleus, dopaminergic neurons of the ventral periaqueductal gray matter, and histaminergic neurons of the tuberomammillary nucleus. Orexin (hypocretin) neurons of the lateral hypothalamic area contribute as well and are thought to have a modulatory influence on the transition between sleep and wakefulness. On the other hand, the sleep system is thought to be controlled by activation of sleep-active cells in the ventrolateral preoptic nucleus (VLPO), which contain the inhibitory neurotransmitters γ-aminobutyric acid and galanin. These cells project to the essential components of the ascending arousal system. Inhibition of the arousal system by the VLPO during sleep is critical for the maintenance and consolidation of sleep.

Antidepressant classes and their receptor profiles are listed in **Table 1**. For definitions of polysomnographic terms, readers are referred to standard scoring manuals.[5]

SELECTIVE SEROTONIN REUPTAKE INHIBITORS
Subjective Effects

Subjective complaints of insomnia and daytime somnolence are common in people with depression being treated with selective serotonin reuptake inhibitors (SSRIs). Of the SSRIs currently indicated for the treatment of depression, fluoxetine's effects on sleep have been the most thoroughly studied. These effects may represent a class effect. Fluoxetine has been found to cause both significant activation and sedation compared with placebo.[6] Rates of activation tend to be stable at dosages between 5 and 40 mg per day, but increase at dosages greater than 40 mg per day. On the other

Table 1
Antidepressant classes and their sleep-related pharmacologic profiles

Medication/Class	Sleep-related Pharmacology	Effects on Sleep Architecture
SSRI	5-HT reuptake inhibition	REM suppression, increased REM latency
SNRI	5-HT, norepinephrine reuptake inhibition	REM suppression, increased REM latency
Trazodone/ nefazodone	5-HT 2 antagonism	Decreased sleep latency, increased SWS
Mirtazapine	5-HT 2 antagonism, H1 antagonism	Decreased sleep latency, increased SWS
TCA	5-HT, norepinephrine reuptake inhibition, H1 antagonism	Decreased sleep latency, REM suppression, increased REM latency

Adapted from Barkoukis TR, Matheson JK, Ferber R, et al, editors. Therapy in sleep medicine. Philadelphia: Elsevier Saunders; 2012.

hand, sedation increases linearly up to dosages of 40 mg per day and then remains stable at dosages between 40 and 60 mg per day. Rates of subjectively reported insomnia and daytime somnolence for various SSRIs are noted in **Fig. 1**.

Polysomnographic Effects

Fluoxetine can cause a decrease in sleep continuity as well as other polysomnographic effects, including REM suppression,[7–10] decreased sleep efficiency,[3,6,11] and increased number of awakenings.[4,7] Disruption in sleep continuity has been found to correlate with plasma levels of fluoxetine and its biologically active metabolite, norfluoxetine. Thus, changes in sleep continuity may develop over time as plasma levels increase because of accumulation of the drug.[3] Fluoxetine also increases the number of oculomotor movements during non-rapid eye movement sleep.[12–14] Although this has not been a consistent finding, it may suggest a generalized increase in central arousal.[15]

SEROTONIN-NOREPINEPHRINE REUPTAKE INHIBITORS
Subjective Effects

Serotonin-norepinephrine reuptake inhibitors (SNRIs) are associated with frequent subjective complaints of insomnia and daytime somnolence as well as vivid dreams. Studies using polysomnography techniques have been limited. Most studies involve the use of the older SNRIs, venlafaxine and duloxetine (**Fig. 2**).

Polysomnographic Effects

Treatment with venlafaxine has been shown to cause an increase in wakefulness after sleep onset (WASO) after 1 month of treatment compared with placebo-treated groups.[16] It significantly increases REM onset latency and reduces total REM time. These effects are evident after 1 week of treatment and persist when monitored for after 1 month of treatment. Treatment with venlafaxine has been associated with periodic limb movements (PLMs), repetitive involuntary movements of the extremities, typically the legs, during sleep or just before falling asleep. These repetitive involuntary movements are polysomnographically recorded as periodic bursts of electromyographic activity in the anterior tibialis electrodes of the lower extremities. The

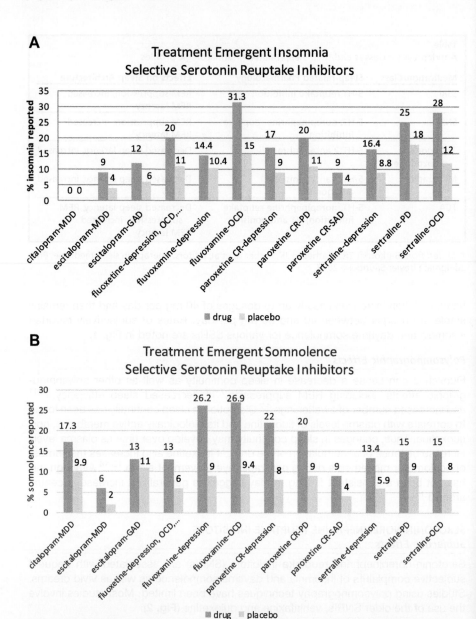

Fig. 1. (*A*, *B*) Complaints of both treatment emergent insomnia and somnolence are common with most SSRIs. Where rates are reported as 0%, the event occurred in less than 2% of patients treated with the medication and at rates less than that with placebo. Caution should be taken in using these figures to predict the incidence of adverse effects in usual clinical practice where conditions and patient characteristics may differ from those in the respective clinical trials. In addition, results are not strictly comparative because they are derived from separate studies performed under differing conditions and with different methodologies. (*Data from* US Food and Drug Administration. FDA Approved Drug Products. Available at: http://www.accessdata.fda.gov/scripts/cder/drugsatfda/index.cfm. Accessed October 2, 2015.)

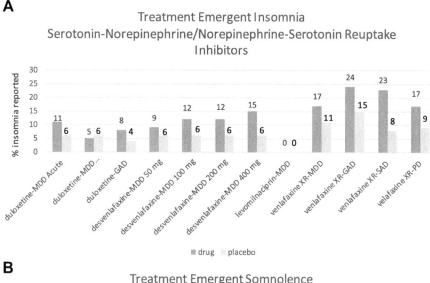

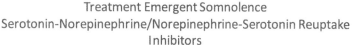

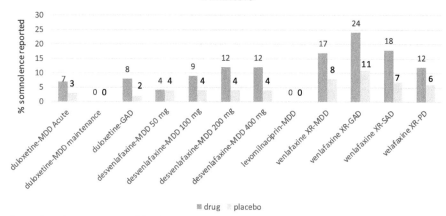

Fig. 2. (*A, B*) Complaints of both treatment emergent insomnia and somnolence are common with most SSRIs/SNRIs. Where rates are reported as 0%, the event occurred in less than 2% of patients treated with the medication and at rates less than that with placebo. Caution should be taken in using these figures to predict the incidence of adverse effects in usual clinical practice where conditions and patient characteristics may differ from those in the respective clinical trials. In addition, results are not strictly comparative because they are derived from separate studies performed under differing conditions and with different methodologies. (*Data from* US Food and Drug Administration. FDA Approved Drug Products. Available at: http://www.accessdata.fda.gov/scripts/cder/drugsatfda/index.cfm. Accessed October 2, 2015.)

pathophysiologic basis of for these movements is unknown, and the basis of the effects of venlafaxine in promoting these movements is also unknown. Effects can be continuous and worsen over time, with rates of greater than 25 PLMs per hour being reported.[17] In some, these movements may persist for up to a week after discontinuation of treatment.

Trazodone

Trazodone's use as an antidepressant is often limited by its tendency to produce daytime somnolence. In that respect, it is often used, at low doses, as a sleep aid or coadministered with an SSRI to decrease the SSRIs' deleterious and disruptive effects on sleep. This effect has not been well studied. When administered alone to depressed patients, trazodone has been shown to increase total sleep time (TST), decrease sleep onset latency (SOL), reduce WASO, increase SWS, and increase REM latency.[18]

Mirtazapine

Daytime somnolence is a common adverse effect of mirtazapine. In clinical trials, up to 54% of patients treated with mirtazapine reported it as an adverse event.[19] However, in practice, this effect can be used to improve sleep disturbances in select populations, although this effect has not been well explored. Mirtazapine produces predominantly antihistaminergic effects at lower doses, compared with increasingly predominant noradrenergic effects at higher doses.[20] Because of this unique pharmacologic profile, mirtazapine is thought to produce relatively more sedation at doses less than 30 mg per day.[21] In depressed patients, it has been shown to significantly increase TST and sleep efficiency and significantly reduce SOL, without significantly altering REM sleep parameters.[22] Although mirtazapine has typically been associated with beneficial effects on sleep, disturbing dreams and confusional states were reported during clinical trials.[23]

Bupropion

Bupropion is associated with reports of insomnia in patients treated for depression and seasonal affective disorder with rates ranging from 11% to 20% depending on the dose, formulation, and condition being treated. However, electroencephalogram studies have shown bupropion to be one of the few antidepressants that actually shortens REM latency and increases total REM sleep time.[24] This finding is in contrast to most other antidepressants, which are prominent suppressants of REM sleep.

New antidepressants

Several medications have recently been approved for the treatment of major depressive disorder (MDD). These medications include levomilnacipran (2013), vilazodone (2011), and vortioxetine (2013). Sleep disturbance was not listed as a common adverse effect in clinical studies for levomilnacipran.[25] Somnolence, insomnia, and abnormal dreams were listed as common adverse effects in clinical trials with vilazodone.[26] Abnormal dreams, but not insomnia or somnolence, were listed as a common adverse effect in clinical trials with vortioxetine.[27] Further studies, including polysomnographic testing in patients taking these medications, are needed to better understand the effects of these newer agents on sleep (**Fig. 3**).

TRICYCLIC ANTIDEPRESSANTS
Subjective Effects

Tertiary amine tricyclic antidepressants (TCAs; amitriptyline, trimipramine) tend to be more sedating, whereas secondary amine TCAs (desipramine, nortriptyline) tend to be more activating. Therefore, it may easier to choose a particular agent in this class that will have the desired effect on sleep profile compared with other classes of antidepressants. Sedating, tertiary amine TCAs tend to shorten SOL, improve sleep continuity and efficiency, and reduce WASO.[28–30] Activating, secondary amine TCAs, on the other hand, tend to prolong SOL, reduce sleep efficiency, and increase WASO.[31] The TCA doxepin, first approved in 1969 for the management of major depression and anxiety and as a topical preparation (5% cream) for pruritus, was recently

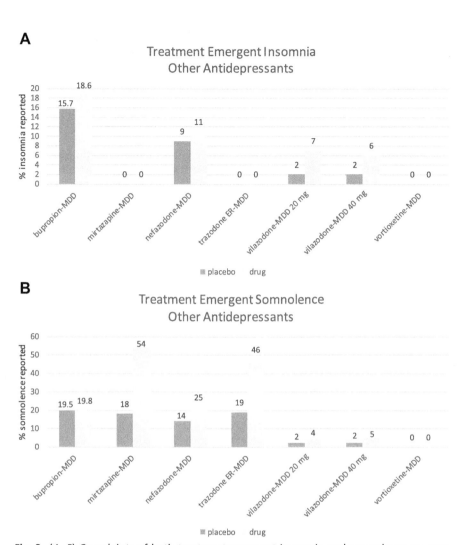

Fig. 3. (*A, B*) Complaints of both treatment emergent insomnia and somnolence are common with most antidepressants. Where rates are reported as 0%, the event occurred in less than 2% of patients treated with the medication and at rates less than that with placebo. Caution should be taken in using these figures to predict the incidence of adverse effects in usual clinical practice where conditions and patient characteristics may differ from those in the respective clinical trials. In addition, results are not strictly comparative because they are derived from separate studies performed under differing conditions and with different methodologies. (*Data from* US Food and Drug Administration. FDA Approved Drug Products. Available at: http://www.accessdata.fda.gov/scripts/cder/drugsatfda/index. cfm. Accessed October 2, 2015.)

reformulated in lower oral doses (3 mg and 6 mg) with demonstrated efficacy for insomnia characterized by difficulties with sleep maintenance following sleep onset.[32] In addition to subjective improvements in insomnia measures, polysomnographic measures of wake after sleep onset, TST, and sleep efficiency have been shown to improve following its administration at bedtime. Although its mechanism of action is not known, it is presumed to promote sleep by antagonizing the histamine-based arousal pathways.[33,34]

Polysomnographic Effects

All TCAs, with the exception of trimipramine, suppress REM sleep; this is manifested by an increase in REM latency and a decreased percentage of time spent in REM sleep.[35–37] At standard antidepressant doses, clomipramine appears to have the most potent REM suppressant effects, although comparative data are limited. Placebo and plasma concentration-controlled studies of maintenance nortriptyline therapy in depressed elderly patients have shown that REM suppression and increased REM latency persist, even in those with no recurrence of depression in 1 year.[38,39] In addition, patients on TCA therapy tend to report intense, vivid dreams, and even nightmares. Recall of dreams may be due to the REM-suppressing effect of the TCA leading to increased pressure for REM.

Monoamine oxidase inhibitors

Treatment with monoamine oxidase inhibitors (MAOIs) is associated with frequent complaints of insomnia, especially with tranylcypromine, which is structurally similar to amphetamine and is more stimulating. MAOIs tend to cause prolonged SOL, impaired sleep continuity, and increased WASO.[40,41] REM suppression is also common, possibly more so with irreversible MAOIs than with reversible MAOIs like moclobemide.[42] REM suppression typically occurs quickly after initiation and persists for months if the medication is continued. REM rebound occurs with discontinuation of therapy and can lead to intense and vivid dreams (**Fig. 4**).

ANTIPSYCHOTICS

Antipsychotics are indicated for the treatment of schizophrenia and other psychotic disorders. Many of the atypical antipsychotics also have indications for the treatment of bipolar disorder and adjunctive treatment of MDDs. Daytime somnolence and sedation seem to be a much more common problem with antipsychotics compared with insomnia. Antipsychotics are thought to exert much of their indicated effects through antagonism of dopamine receptors. Many typical and atypical antipsychotics also exert effects on various monoamines as well as histamine and muscarinic cholinergic receptors. These effects may increase the likelihood of somnolence and can also alter certain polysomnogram (PSG) sleep parameters (**Table 2**).

Typical Antipsychotics

Studies evaluating the effects of typical antipsychotic drugs in patients with schizophrenia are limited. Of the studies that are available,[43–45] haloperidol, thiothixene, and flupentixol possibly reduce stage 2 sleep latency, increase TST and sleep efficiency, and significantly increase REM latency. SWS seems to remain unaffected. Validity of these results, however, is diminished by methodological problems and the limited number of studies.

Atypical Antipsychotics

Quetiapine, which is approved for the treatment of schizophrenia, acute depressive, manic, and mixed episodes of bipolar I disorder, and as adjunct treatment of MDD, exhibits strong histamine (H1)-receptor antagonism and moderate affinity for 5-hydroxytryptamine (5-HT) serotonin type 2A receptors.[46] Antagonism at these sites is thought to be responsible for quetiapine's sedative effects.

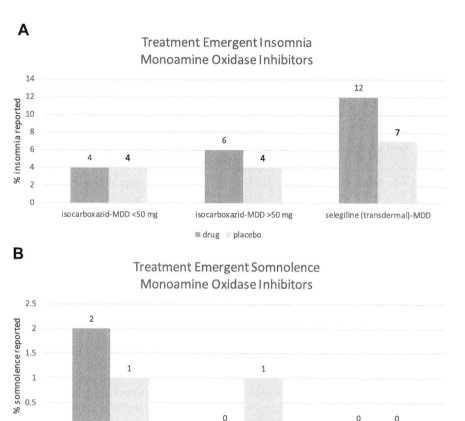

Fig. 4. (*A*, *B*) Complaints of both treatment emergent insomnia and somnolence are common with most MAOIs. Where rates are reported as 0%, the event occurred in less than 2% of patients treated with the medication and at rates less than that with placebo. Caution should be taken in using these figures to predict the incidence of adverse effects in usual clinical practice where conditions and patient characteristics may differ from those in the respective clinical trials. In addition, results are not strictly comparative because they are derived from separate studies performed under differing conditions and with different methodologies. (*Data from* US Food and Drug Administration. FDA Approved Drug Products. Available at: http://www.accessdata.fda.gov/scripts/cder/drugsatfda/index.cfm. Accessed October 2, 2015.)

In a meta-analysis of the numbers needed to treat to harm (NNTH) for discontinuation due to sedation,[47] both quetiapine-IR 300 mg per day and 600 mg per day resulted in significant risk of sedation with NNTH of 8 for both doses in patients with bipolar depression. NNTH with quetiapine-XR 150 mg per day and 300 mg per day in patients with refractory MDD were 9 and 7, respectively. NNTH with quetiapine-XR 50 mg per day, 150 mg per day, and 300 mg per day in patients with nonrefractory MDD were 5, 3, and 4, respectively.

In an open-label pilot study,[48] 18 adults with insomnia were treated with quetiapine 25 mg at bedtime, with dosages being increased to 50 mg in 7 patients and 75 mg in 1 patient. There were improvements in subjective and objective sleep parameters after

Table 2
Antipsychotic classes and their sleep-related pharmacologic profiles

Medication/Class	Sleep-related Pharmacology	Effects on Sleep Architecture
Typical antipsychotics	Dopamine 2 receptor antagonism, H 1 antagonism, anticholinergic	Increased TST, improved sleep efficiency, decreased SOL, decreased WASO, unaffected SWS, increased REM latency
Atypical antipsychotics	Dopamine 2 receptor antagonism, 5-HT 2 antagonism, H 1 antagonism	Increased TST, increased sleep efficiency, decreased SOL, decreased WASO, increased SWS

Adapted from Barkoukis TR, Matheson JK, Ferber R, et al, editors. Therapy in sleep medicine. Philadelphia: Elsevier Saunders; 2012.

2 weeks that continued at 6 weeks. TST and sleep efficiency evaluated by polysomnography were significantly improved at 2 and 6 weeks. Pittsburgh Sleep Quality Index (PSQI) scores and subscores were also statistically improved at 2 and 6 weeks. Transient morning hangover was noted as a frequently reported adverse effect.

In non-PSG-based studies in patients with posttraumatic stress disorder, relatively low doses of quetiapine were associated with improvement in the PSQI global sleep score: sleep quality was subjectively better; SOL was reduced; TST improved; and episodes of terror and acting out dreams were reduced.[49]

In patients with schizophrenia, clozapine, which is sedating, has been noted to reduce SOL and increase TST and sleep efficiency.[50] In a population of treatment-refractory patients with bipolar disorder, the average time of going to bed was 55 minutes earlier with clozapine compared with that reported at baseline.[51] Similarly, risperidone has been shown to improve sleep maintenance and to decrease WASO in patients with schizophrenia.[52]

A 14-day PSG study evaluating the effects of paliperidone ER was conducted in a group of patients with schizophrenia-related insomnia.[53] In this double-blind, randomized, placebo-controlled study, paliperidone ER resulted in clinically and statistically significant differences in sleep measurements from baseline. There were significant reductions in SOL, WASO, time awake in bed, and stage 1 sleep duration. In addition, there was a prolongation of TST, stage 2 sleep duration, and REM sleep duration, and an increase in sleep efficiency index. Compared with placebo, paliperidone ER did not exacerbate daytime somnolence. Overall, it was well tolerated and improved sleep architecture and sleep continuity in this group of patients with schizophrenia and concomitant insomnia.

PSG studies in patients treated with olanzapine have shown significant decreases in wake time and stage 1 sleep and significant increases in TST, stage 2 sleep, and SWS (**Fig. 5**).[54,55]

RESTLESS LEGS SYNDROME

Antipsychotic agents may cause or exacerbate RLS.[50] A case series of 7 patients given low-dose quetiapine reported a dose-dependent provocation of RLS.[56] The investigators noted that most of these patients suffered from affective disorders and were on concomitant antidepressants. The Prescribing Information for quetiapine notes the occurrence of restless legs syndrome (RLS) in 2% of persons on quetiapine versus none on placebo.[57] Other case reports also seem to suggest that patients with affective disorders who are taking antidepressants may be particularly susceptible to

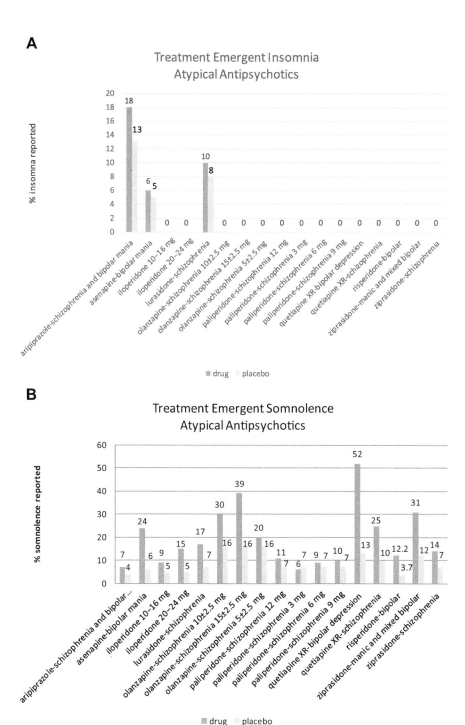

A

Treatment Emergent Insomnia Atypical Antipsychotics

■ drug ■ placebo

B

Treatment Emergent Somnolence Atypical Antipsychotics

■ drug ■ placebo

Fig. 5. (*A, B*) Complaints of treatment emergent somnolence are common with most antipsychotics. Caution should be taken in using these figures to predict the incidence of adverse effects in usual clinical practice where conditions and patient characteristics may differ from those in the respective clinical trials. In addition, results are not strictly comparative because they are derived from separate studies performed under differing conditions and with different methodologies. (*Data from* US Food and Drug Administration. FDA Approved Drug Products. Available at: http://www.accessdata.fda.gov/scripts/cder/drugsatfda/index.cfm. Accessed October 2, 2015.)

the development of RLS. Antidepressant-induced RLS is most likely to occur with mirtazapine, which can be associated with provoking or deteriorating RLS in 28% of patients.[58] Antidepressant-induced RLS typically occurs within the first few days of treatment. Antidepressants are more likely to be associated with RLS in men than in women.[59]

It has been suggested that RLS is related to the dopaminergic effects of antidepressants.[60] These investigators suggested sertraline may be least likely among the SSRIs to cause RLS because it blocks dopamine reuptake. Bupropion may reduce RLS by increasing dopaminergic activity.[61]

NONBENZODIAZEPINE HYPNOTICS

Parasomnias like sleepwalking and sleep-related eating disorders (SRED) have been reported with nonbenzodiazepine hypnotics. In a review of parasomnias in psychiatric outpatients,[62] sleepwalking was linked to zolpidem and zopiclone, whereas both sleepwalking and SRED were associated with zolpidem alone. Parasomnias with this class of medication were more likely in patients taking them regularly rather than on an as-needed basis.

STIMULANTS

Stimulants are commonly prescribed for the treatment of attention-deficit/hyperactivity disorder (ADHD). The relationship between sleep and medication in children with ADHD is complex. Insomnia or delayed SOL greater than 30 minutes is one of the most common adverse effects associated with stimulant medications.[63] However, the effects of methylphenidate on sleep may depend on the length of time the child has been on the medication.[64] In addition, there are reports of children having difficulty falling asleep when the medication is being weaned off as well as children who fall asleep easily after taking a low dose of medication.[65] Results of polysomnographic studies in children with ADHD who were receiving methylphenidate have been inconsistent.[66]

SUMMARY

Antidepressant and antipsychotic agents frequently result in sleep-related adverse effects, primarily insomnia and daytime somnolence. However, these effects have not been well evaluated. Data from placebo-controlled trials are available primarily in the form of spontaneous reports rather than systematic assessments. Where sleep-related effects have been specifically studied as end points, the data are limited to small sample sizes and with methodological inconsistencies. In addition, comparative data between various agents are lacking. Nevertheless, the data available do provide some guidance regarding possible adverse effects on sleep and wakefulness, so that a therapeutic plan can be crafted for each patient's individual clinical situation.

REFERENCES

1. Benca RM, Obermeyer WH, Thisted RA, et al. Sleep and psychiatric disorders. A meta-analysis. Arch Gen Psychiatry 1992;49(8):651–68.

2. Pratt LA, Brody DJ, Gu Q. Antidepressant Use in Persons Aged 12 and Over: United States, 2005–2008. Hyattsville (MD): U.S. Department of Health and Human Services; Centers for Disease Control and Prevention; 2011. Available at: http://www.cdc.gov/nchs/data/databriefs/db76.pdf.

3. Saper CB, Scammell TE, Lu J. Hypothalamic regulation of sleep and circadian rhythms. Nature 2005;437(7063):1257–63.

4. Fuller PM, Gooley JJ, Saper CB. Neurobiology of the sleep-wake cycle: sleep architecture, circadian regulation, and regulatory feedback. J Biol Rhythms 2006; 21(6):482–93.

5. Berry RB, Brooks R, Gamaldo CE, et al, for the American Academy of Sleep Medicine. The AASM manual for the scoring of sleep and associated events: rules, terminology and technical specifications, version 2.2. Darien (IL): American Academy of Sleep Medicine; 2015. Available at: www.aasmnet.org.

6. Beasley CM Jr, Sayler ME, Weiss AM, et al. Fluoxetine: activating and sedating effects at multiple fixed doses. J Clin Psychopharmacol 1992;12(5):328–33.

7. Armitage R, Rush AJ, Trivedi M, et al. The effects of nefazodone on sleep architecture in depression. Neuropsychopharmacology 1994;10(2):123–7.

8. Kerkhofs M, Rielaert C, De Maertelaer V, et al. Fluoxetine in major depression: efficacy, safety and effects on sleep polygraphic variables. Int Clin Psychopharmacol 1990;5:253–60.

9. Hendrickse WA, Roffwarg HP, Grannemann BD, et al. The effects of fluoxetine on the polysomnogram of depressed outpatients: a pilot study. Neuropsychopharmacology 1994;10(2):85–91.

10. Gillin JC, Rapaport M, Erman MK, et al. A comparison of nefazodone and fluoxetine on mood and on objective, subjective, and clinician-rated measures of sleep in depressed patients: a double-blind, 8-week clinical trial. J Clin Psychiatry 1997;58(5):185–92.

11. Trivedi MH, Rush AJ, Armitage R, et al. Effects of fluoxetine on the polysomnogram in outpatients with major depression. Neuropsychopharmacology 1999; 20(5):447–59.

12. Keck PE Jr, Hudson JI, Dorsey CM, et al. Effect of fluoxetine on sleep. Biol Psychiatry 1991;29(6):618–9.

13. Schenck CH, Mahowald MW, Kim SW, et al. Prominent eye movements during NREM sleep and REM sleep behavior disorder associated with fluoxetine treatment of depression and obsessive-compulsive disorder. Sleep 1992;15(3): 226–35.

14. Dorsey CM, Lukas SE, Cunningham SL. Fluoxetine-induced sleep disturbance in depressed patients. Neuropsychopharmacology 1996;14(6):437–42.

15. Vasar V, Appelberg B, Rimon R, et al. The effect of fluoxetine on sleep: a longitudinal, double-blind polysomnographic study of healthy volunteers. Int Clin Psychopharmacol 1994;9(3):203–6.

16. Luthringer R, Toussaint M, Schaltenbrand N, et al. A double-blind, placebo-controlled evaluation of the effects of orally administered venlafaxine on sleep in inpatients with major depression. Psychopharmacol Bull 1996;32(4):637–46.

17. Salin-Pascual RJ, Galicia-Polo L, Drucker-Colin R. Sleep changes after 4 consecutive days of venlafaxine administration in normal volunteers. J Clin Psychiatry 1997;58(8):348–50.

18. Mouret J, Lemoine P, Minuit MP, et al. Effects of trazodone on the sleep of depressed subjects–a polygraphic study. Psychopharmacology 1988; 95(Suppl):S37–43.

19. Organon, Inc. Remeron—a novel pharmacological treatment for depression. West Orange (NJ): Organon, Inc; 1996.

20. Kent JM. SNaRIs, NaSSAs, and NaRIs: new agents for the treatment of depression. Lancet (London, England) 2000;355(9207):911–8.

21. Grasmader K, Verwohlt PL, Kuhn KU, et al. Relationship between mirtazapine dose, plasma concentration, response, and side effects in clinical practice. Pharmacopsychiatry 2005;38(3):113–7.

22. Winokur A, Sateia MJ, Hayes JB, et al. Acute effects of mirtazapine on sleep continuity and sleep architecture in depressed patients: a pilot study. Biol Psychiatry 2000;48(1):75–8.

23. Organon USA. Product information REMERON oral tablets, mirtazapine tablets. Roseland (NJ): Organon USA, Inc; 2007.

24. Nofzinger EA, Reynolds CF 3rd, Thase ME, et al. REM sleep enhancement by bupropion in depressed men. Am J Psychiatry 1995;152(2):274–6.

25. Forest Pharmaceuticals USA, Inc. Product information for FETZIMA (levomilnacipran) extended-release capsules. St Louis (MO): Forest Pharmaceuticals USA, Inc; 2013.

26. Forest Pharmaceuticals USA, Inc. Product information for VIIBRYD (vilazodone hydrochloride) tablets. Cincinnati (OH): Forest Pharmaceuticals USA, Inc; 2015.

27. Takeda Pharmaceuticals America, Inc. Product information for BRINTELLIX (vortioxetine) tablets. Deerfield (IL): Takeda Pharmaceuticals America, Inc; 2013.

28. Kupfer DJ, Spiker DG, Rossi A, et al. Nortriptyline and EEG sleep in depressed patients. Biol Psychiatry 1982;17(5):535–46.

29. Shipley JE, Kupfer DJ, Dealy RS, et al. Differential effects of amitriptyline and of zimelidine on the sleep electroencephalogram of depressed patients. Clin Pharmacol Ther 1984;36(2):251–9.

30. Ware JC, Brown FW, Moorad PJ Jr, et al. Effects on sleep: a double-blind study comparing trimipramine to imipramine in depressed insomniac patients. Sleep 1989;12(6):537–49.

31. Kupfer DJ, Perel JM, Pollock BG, et al. Fluvoxamine versus desipramine: Comparative polysomnographic effects. Biol Psychiatry 1991;29(1):23–40.

32. Markov D, Doghramji K. Doxepin for insomnia. Curr Psychiatry 2010;9(10):67–77.

33. Roth T, Rogowski R, Hull S, et al. Efficacy and safety of doxepin 1 mg, 3 mg, and 6 mg in adults with primary insomnia. Sleep 2007;30(11):1555–61.

34. Scharf M, Rogowski R, Hull S, et al. Efficacy and safety of doxepin 1 mg, 3 mg, and 6 mg in elderly patients with primary insomnia: a randomized, double-blind, placebo controlled crossover study. J Clin Psychiatry 2008;69:1557–64.

35. Vogel GW, Buffenstein A, Minter K, et al. Drug effects on REM sleep and on endogenous depression. Neurosci Biobehav Rev 1990;14(1):49–63.

36. Nofzinger EA, Schwartz RM, Reynolds CF 3rd, et al. Affect intensity and phasic REM sleep in depressed men before and after treatment with cognitive-behavioral therapy. J Consult Clin Psychol 1994;62(1):83–91.

37. Sharpley AL, Cowen PJ. Effect of pharmacologic treatments on the sleep of depressed patients. Biol Psychiatry 1995;37(2):85–98.

38. Reynolds CF 3rd, Buysse DJ, Brunner DP, et al. Maintenance nortriptyline effects on electroencephalographic sleep in elderly patients with recurrent major depression: double-blind, placebo- and plasma-level-controlled evaluation. Biol Psychiatry 1997;42(7):560–7.

39. Taylor MP, Reynolds CF 3rd, Frank E, et al. EEG sleep measures in later-life bereavement depression. A randomized, double-blind, placebo-controlled evaluation of nortriptyline. Am J Geriatr Psychiatry 1999;7(1):41–7.

40. Wyatt RJ, Fram DH, Kupfer DJ, et al. Total prolonged drug-induced REM sleep suppression in anxious-depressed patients. Arch Gen Psychiatry 1971;24(2):145–55.

41. Kupfer DJ, Bowers MB Jr. REM sleep and central monoamine oxidase inhibition. Psychopharmacologia 1972;27(3):183–90.

42. Monti JM. Effect of a reversible monoamine oxidase-A inhibitor (moclobemide) on sleep of depressed patients. Br J Psychiatry Suppl 1989;(6):61–5.

43. Wetter TC, Lauer CJ, Gillich G, et al. The electroencephalographic sleep pattern in schizophrenic patients treated with clozapine or classical antipsychotic drugs. J Psychiatr Res 1996;30(6):411–9.

44. Hinze-Selch D, Mullington J, Orth A, et al. Effects of clozapine on sleep: a longitudinal study. Biol Psychiatry 1997;42(4):260–6.

45. Touyz SW, Saayman GS, Zabow T. A psychophysiological investigation of the long-term effects of clozapine upon sleep patterns of normal young adults. Psychopharmacology 1978;56(1):69–73.

46. Stahl SM. Selective histamine H1 antagonism: novel hypnotic and pharmacologic actions challenge classical notions of antihistamines. CNS Spectr 2008;13:1027–38.

47. Gao K, Kemp DE, Fein E, et al. Number needed to treat to harm for discontinuation due to adverse events in the treatment of bipolar depression, major depressive disorder, and generalized anxiety disorder with atypical antipsychotics. J Clin Psychiatry 2011;72(8):1063–71.

48. Wiegand MH, Landry F, Bruckner T, et al. Quetiapine in primary insomnia: a pilot study. Psychopharmacology 2008;196(2):337–8.

49. Robert S, Hamner MB, Kose S, et al. Quetiapine improves sleep disturbances in combat veterans with PTSD: sleep data from a prospective, open-label study. J Clin Psychopharmacol 2005;25(4):387–8.

50. Krystal AD, Goforth HW, Roth T. Effects of antipsychotic medications on sleep in schizophrenia. Int Clin Psychopharmacol 2008;23(3):150–60.

51. Armitage R, Cole D, Suppes T, et al. Effects of clozapine on sleep in bipolar and schizoaffective disorders. Prog NeuroPsychopharmacol Biol Psychiatry 2004;28(7):1065–70.

52. Dursun SM, Patel JK, Burke JG, et al. Effects of typical antipsychotic drugs and risperidone on the quality of sleep in patients with schizophrenia: a pilot study. J Psychiatry Neurosci 1999;24(4):333–7.

53. Luthringer R, Staner L, Noel N, et al. A double-blind, placebo-controlled, randomized study evaluating the effect of paliperidone extended-release tablets on sleep architecture in patients with schizophrenia. Int Clin Psychopharmacol 2007;22(5):299–308.

54. Sharpley AL, Vassallo CM, Cowen PJ. Olanzapine increases slow-wave sleep: Evidence for blockade of central 5-HT(2C) receptors in vivo. Biol Psychiatry 2000;47(5):468–70.

55. Salin-Pascual RJ, Herrera-Estrella M, Galicia-Polo L, et al. Olanzapine acute administration in schizophrenic patients increases delta sleep and sleep efficiency. Biol Psychiatry 1999;46(1):141–3.

56. Rittmannsberger H, Werl R. Restless legs syndrome induced by quetiapine: report of seven cases and review of the literature. Int J Neuropsychopharmacol 2013;16:1427–31.

57. AstraZeneca Pharmaceuticals LP. Product information for SEROQUEL (quetiapine fumarate) tablets. Wilmington (DE): AstraZeneca Pharmaceuticals LP; 2009.

58. Rottach KG, Schaner BM, Kirch MH, et al. Restless legs syndrome as side effect of second generation antidepressants. J Psychiatr Res 2008;43(1):70–5.

59. Baughman KR, Bourguet CC, Ober SK. Gender differences in the association be-
    tween antidepressant use and restless legs syndrome. Mov Disord 2009;24(7):
    1054–9.
60. Perroud N, Lazignac C, Baleydier B, et al. Restless legs syndrome induced by
    citalopram: a psychiatric emergency? Gen Hosp Psychiatry 2007;29(1):72–4.
61. Kim SW, Shin IS, Kim JM, et al. Bupropion may improve restless legs syndrome: a
    report of three cases. Clin Neuropharmacol 2005;28(6):298–301.
62. Lam SP, Fong SY, Ho CK, et al. Parasomnia among psychiatric outpatients: a clin-
    ical, epidemiologic, cross-sectional study. J Clin Psychiatry 2008;69(9):1374–82.
63. Stein MA. Unravelling sleep problems in treated and untreated children with
    ADHD. J Child Adolesc Psychopharmacol 1999;9(3):157–68.
64. Wigal SB, Wong AA, Jun A, et al. Adverse events in medication treatment-naive
    children with attention-deficit/hyperactivity disorder: results from a small,
    controlled trial of lisdexamfetamine dimesylate. J Child Adolesc Psychopharma-
    col 2012;22(2):149–56.
65. Chatoor I, Wells KC, Conners CK, et al. The effects of nocturnally administered
    stimulant medication on EEG sleep and behavior in hyperactive children. J Am
    Acad Child Psychiatry 1983;22(4):337–42.
66. Sadeh A, Pergamin L, Bar-Haim Y. Sleep in children with attention-deficit hyper-
    activity disorder: a meta-analysis of polysomnographic studies. Sleep Med Rev
    2006;10(6):381–98.

Antidepressants and Suicidality

David A. Brent, MD

KEYWORDS

- Depression • Antidepressant • Suicide • Suicidal events • Adolescents
- Young adults • Clinical trials

KEY POINTS

- Second-generation antidepressants are associated with a slightly increased risk for suicidal events compared with placebo in randomized clinical trials (RCTs) in youth.
- Four to eleven times more depressed youth benefit from antidepressants than experience a suicidal event.
- Pharmacoepidemiologic studies, which are much larger and more representative of patient populations than RCTs, show a protective effect of regional antidepressant use on suicide.
- Youth most likely to experience a suicidal event have high baseline suicidal ideation, family conflict, alcohol and substance use, nonsuicidal self-injury, and non-response to treatment.
- The clinician can mitigate suicidal risk in depressed youths through education, a safety plan, close clinical monitoring, targeting of suicidal risk factors, and rational dosing.

DEFINITIONS OF SELF-HARM

The definitions of self-harm used in this article are provided in **Table 1**.[1]

META-ANALYSES OF RANDOMIZED CLINICAL TRIALS

Hammad and colleagues[2] first reported, in a meta-analysis of 24 randomized clinical trials (RCTs) (20 of which had data on suicidal events), that antidepressant use was associated with an increased risk for suicidal events in depressed youth (odds ratio [OR] = 1.66) and across indications (OR = 1.95). A subsequent meta-analysis of RCTs registered by the Food and Drug Administration (FDA) across the life span showed an increased rate of suicidal events in adults younger than 25 (OR = 1.62), but a protective effect in those aged 25 to 64 (OR = 0.87) and older than 65 (OR = 0.37).[3] A meta-analysis of 27 youth antidepressant RCTs found an increased rate of suicidal events with a risk-difference of 0.7% (meaning the rate of suicidal events in the medication group was higher than the placebo group by

Western Psychiatric Institute & Clinic, 3811 O'Hara Street, BFT 311, Pittsburgh, PA 15213, USA
E-mail address: brentda@upmc.edu

Psychiatr Clin N Am 39 (2016) 503–512
http://dx.doi.org/10.1016/j.psc.2016.04.002   **psych.theclinics.com**

Table 1	
Definitions of self-harm outcomes	
Type of Self-Harm	**Definition**
Suicidal ideation	Thoughts of death, thoughts of one's own death, with or without intent or a plan
Suicide attempt	Self-destructive behavior with explicit or inferred intent to die
Nonsuicidal self-harm	Self-destructive behavior with an aim to modify negative affect, punish self, or escape, but without any suicidal intent
Suicide	Suicide attempt that results in a fatality
Suicidal event	New-onset or worsened suicidal ideation or suicidal behavior

Adapted from Posner K, Oquendo MA, Gould M, et al. Columbia classification algorithm of suicide assessment (C-CASA): classification of suicidal events in the FDA's pediatric suicidal risk analysis of antidepressants. Am J Psychiatry 2007;164(7):1035–43.

0.7%), with a 1.7-fold increase in suicidal events (**Fig. 1**).[4] In addition, 11 times more depressed adolescents responded to an antidepressant than experienced a suicidal event, with even higher benefit-risk ratios for those with obsessive compulsive or anxiety disorders. A Cochrane review of adolescent depression RCTs found similarly increased risks for suicidal events (OR = 1.6), with approximately 4.5 times the number of youth attaining clinical remission as experienced suicidal events.[5]

WHY IS THERE AN INCREASED RISK FOR SUICIDAL EVENTS FOUND IN THOSE YOUNGER THAN 25?

1. There are no proven explanations, but the following are commonly offered: Antidepressant treatment in the young is more likely to uncover a proclivity to bipolar disorder, induce a possible mixed state, and thereby increase the risk for suicide.[6] The younger the patient treated with an antidepressant, the higher the risk for antidepressant-associated mania (**Fig. 2**).[7] One meta-analysis estimated that the risk of mania in depressed youth treated with an antidepressant versus placebo was 10% versus 0.45%.[8]

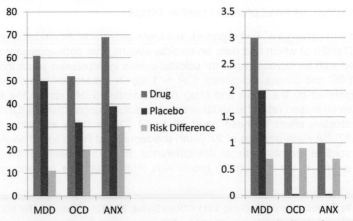

Fig. 1. Risks and benefits of antidepressants by indication in youth. (*Data from* Bridge JA, Iyengar S, Salary CB, et al. Clinical response and risk for reported suicidal ideation and suicide attempts in pediatric antidepressant treatment: a meta-analysis of randomized controlled trials. JAMA 2007;297(15):1683–96.)

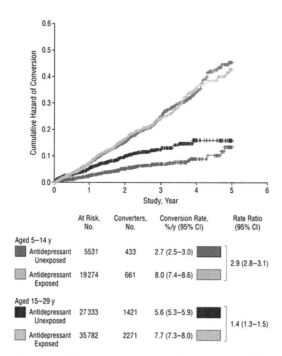

Fig. 2. Risk of mania and antidepressant treatment by age. CI, confidence interval. (*From* Martin A, Young C, Leckman JF, et al. Age effects on antidepressant-induced manic conversion. Arch Pediatr Adolesc Med 2004;158(8):777; with permission.)

2. Developmental differences associated with the transition from adolescence to adulthood may explain the differential adverse effects of antidepressants. A lack of maturity in prefrontal myelination that could predispose to impulsivity,[9] and higher densities of 5HT1A and 5HT2A serotonergic receptors have been reported in younger individuals.[10,11] Higher density of 5HT1A receptors is associated with higher lethality suicide attempts[12] and nonresponse to a selective serotonin reuptake inhibitor (SSRI),[13] whereas greater 5HT2A density has been associated with impulsive aggression,[14] a key risk factor for youth suicide.[15]

3. Younger patients metabolize antidepressants more quickly. For example, at lower doses of sertraline, its half-life is much shorter in adolescents than in adults.[16] This may be important because greater drug concentration may be related to a greater likelihood of response, and in drugs with shorter half-lives, lower doses in adolescents may be associated with experience of withdrawal symptoms.[17] Among 7 antidepressants studied in adolescent depression, there is a high inverse correlation (rho = −0.79) between the half-life of the drug and the rate of suicidal events in those studies.[18] However, suicidal events are also seen in patients treated with fluoxetine, which has a half-life of approximately 5 days and whose active metabolite, norfluoxetine, has a half-life of approximately 15 days.

4. Suicidal events are more tightly tied to depression in older adults, whereas in younger individuals, substance abuse and impulsive aggression make a stronger contribution.[15] In meta-analyses of RCTs of fluoxetine, a similar decline in depressive symptoms is seen in adolescents and in adults, but a decline in suicidal ideation, and its correlation with a decline in depression was observed only in adults.[19]

This may explain why antidepressants are found to be protective against suicidal events only in older adults.[3]

5. Antidepressants may worsen sleep.[20] Insomnia is one of the most potent risk factors for suicidal behavior.[21]

WHAT IS THE CLINICAL SIGNIFICANCE OF SUICIDAL EVENTS?

Every increase in suicidal ideation should be taken seriously, but to provide clinical context, in adolescent RCTs of adolescent depression, of 80 suicidal events, most (46/80, 57.5%) were increases in suicidal ideation, rather than preparatory behavior for a suicide attempt, or actual attempts. Moreover, in nearly all RCTs, suicidal events were assessed by spontaneous report from patients, rather than by systematic assessment, a method that underestimates the number of true events by more than twofold.[22] It has been posited that suicidal events in patients treated with medication may be more likely to come to clinical attention than those treated with placebo, because medication-treated patients may have other adverse effects that result in greater clinical scrutiny.[23]

PHARMACOEPIDEMIOLOGIC STUDIES

Most pharmacoepidemiologic studies find a relationship between greater number of sales or prescriptions of antidepressants and a lower suicide rate. An inverse relationship between sales of SSRIs and suicide has been found in 24 countries, with the strongest findings among youth younger than 25 (**Fig. 3**).[24] There is also an inverse relationship between prescriptions of SSRIs and suicide in a county-by-county analysis in the United States.[25] This relationship was found only for SSRI prescriptions; the higher the proportion of tricyclic antidepressant prescriptions of the total antidepressants prescribed, the higher the suicide rate.[25] In the period from 1990 to 2000, it was found that for every 1% increase in antidepressant prescriptions, there was a drop in the suicide rate of 0.23 per 100,000.[26] A propensity-matching study in 24,119 depressed adolescents found no increased risk for a suicide attempt in those who started taking an antidepressant, and found that longer duration of treatment (>180 days) was protective against suicide attempts relative to shorter treatment (<55 days).[27] A prospective follow-up of a Finnish cohort of 15,390 hospitalized suicide attempters found that SSRI use was associated with a higher rate of suicide

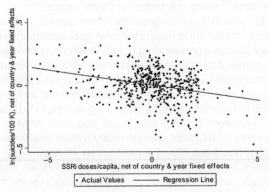

Fig. 3. Antidepressants, suicides, and drug regulation. (*From* Ludwig J, Marcotte DE. Anti-depressants, suicide, and drug regulation. J Policy Anal Manage 2005;24(2):259; with permission.)

attempts but a lower rate of suicide in both adolescents and adults.[28] A longitudinal study of antidepressant prescription in a Dutch sample found no overall association between prescriptions and suicidal behavior, although there was an increased rate of suicide on the first day of initiation of medication and in the fourth week of treatment.[29]

Some of the association between antidepressant use and suicide attempt in cross-sectional studies may be due to confounding of indication and treatment. In a large group health maintenance organization (HMO), the most common event *preceding* the initiation of an antidepressant was a suicide attempt.[30] The rate of attempts subsequent to the initiation of an antidepressant was much lower than the rate before the initiation (**Fig. 4**). Similarly, one large propensity-matching study of 221,028 adolescents found that there was a strong association between antidepressant use and suicide attempt that disappeared after adjustment for clinical confounders.[31] One propensity-matched, prospective case-control study has found an increased risk of suicide and suicide attempt in young individuals associated with antidepressant treatment.[32] However, this finding is inconsistent with the very low rate (<10%) of positive toxicologies for antidepressants found in adolescent suicide postmortem samples.[33] Other studies have found an association with the use of higher doses of antidepressants and suicidal behavior regardless of age, although these associations could be explained by the use of higher doses in those with more refractory conditions.[34,35]

WHY ARE THE FINDINGS OF PHARMACOEPIDEMIOLOGIC STUDIES SO DIFFERENT FROM THOSE OF RCTs?

First, RCTs routinely exclude those at high suicidal risk, such as those patients with a recent suicide attempt. Conversely, a suicide attempt is one of the most common reasons to initiate antidepressants.[30,31] Therefore, RCTs are not informative about the effect of antidepressants on patients at high suicidal risk. Second, the sample size of pharmacoepidemiologic studies is much larger, and the time frame much

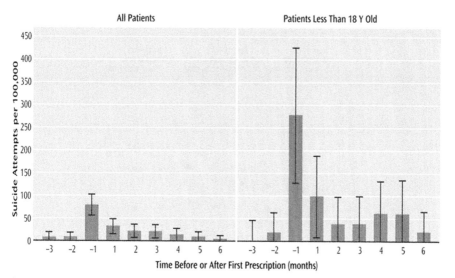

Fig. 4. Rates of suicide attempts during the 3 months before and the 6 months after initial antidepressant prescription. (*From* Simon GE, Savarino J, Operskalski B, et al. Suicide risk during antidepressant treatment. Am J Psychiatry 2006;163(1):44; with permission.)

longer compared with RCTs, providing sufficient power to detect differences in completed suicide rather than just effects on suicidal events. Third, although RCTs allow for tight experimental control and comparability of those treated with medication versus placebo, pharmacoepidemiologic studies can use propensity matching or statistical adjustment for confounders to avoid confounding indication with outcome.

THE BLACK BOX WARNING AS NATURAL EXPERIMENT

In 2004, the FDA issued a warning affixed to all antidepressants about the risk of suicidal events associated with antidepressants in youth. In comparing the period before versus after the so-called Black Box Warning, there were drops in antidepressant prescriptions for youth in the Netherlands, the United States, Canada, and the United Kingdom,[36–39] accompanied by decline in the rate of diagnosis of depressive disorders (**Fig. 5**),[37] number of visits for the treatment of depressive disorders,[38] and increases in suicide in all the previously noted countries but the United Kingdom.[36,38–40] Trends before and after the Black Box Warning in one large group HMO, found a decline in antidepressant use of 31.0% in adolescents and 24.3% in young adults, with a similar magnitude of increase in psychotropic drug overdoses. The study has been criticized insofar as overdoses of psychotropic agents do not include all of suicidal behavior and could be confounded by the presence of psychiatric disorder in patients or their family members. However, if antidepressants were a true risk factor for suicidal behavior, one might have expected a *decline* in overdoses, not an increase.

IN WHOM ARE SUICIDAL EVENTS MOST LIKELY TO OCCUR?

In the major RCTs for adolescent depression, suicidal events were most likely to occur in those who showed nonsuicidal self-injury, high suicidal ideation, family conflict, drug or alcohol abuse, and treatment nonresponse.[22,40,41] The addition of cognitive behavior therapy (CBT) to antidepressant treatment was protective against suicidal events in some, but not other studies.[42] Starting depressed adolescents or young

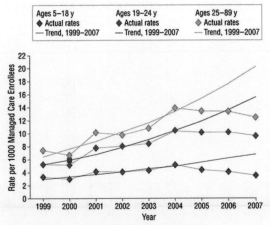

Fig. 5. PHARMetrics patient-centric database population rates of major depressive disorder (actual and predicted) by age group (male and female individuals combined). (*From* Libby AM, Orton HD, Valuck RJ. Persisting decline in depression treatment after FDA warnings. Arch Gen Psychiatry 2009;66(6):635; with permission.)

adults at a higher than usual antidepressant dose (eg, the equivalent of fluoxetine 40 mg/d) may also increase the risk of self-harm.[43] In children and adolescents, the extant trials do not provide sufficient power to determine if suicidal events are more commonly associated with specific antidepressants. The risk-difference (% difference in rate of suicidal events on drug vs placebo) for suicidal events was highest in venlafaxine (4), intermediate for fluoxetine (2), and lower for mirtazapine (1), escitalopram (0), and citalopram (−1).[4] Larger studies that include young adults, but not adolescents have found no difference in the rates of suicidal events across SSRIs,[35,44] but higher rates of suicide in mirtazapine relative to citalopram, and higher rates of suicide attempt and self-harm in venlafaxine, mirtazapine, and trazodone, relative to citalopram.[35] In the latter study, the differential effects of these drugs on suicide and suicidal behavior appeared to be stronger in older subgroups.

HOW CAN CLINICIANS MINIMIZE THE RISK FOR SUICIDAL EVENTS WHEN USING ANTIDEPRESSANTS?

Education

Clinicians should educate patients younger than 25, and the parents of children and adolescents, about the possible adverse effects of antidepressants, such as mania, agitation, akathisia, sleep difficulties, and withdrawal symptoms, all of which could increase the risk for suicidal ideation and behavior. Clinicians should elicit sources of hopelessness about the effects of treatment, and instill realistic hope about the likelihood of achieving symptomatic relief. In addition, clinicians should explain to families that there is a small, but real increased risk for suicidal ideation and behavior in clinical trials, but that the number of youth who benefit from treatment is much greater than the number who experience events.[45]

Close Monitoring During Initiation of Treatment and Dose Changes

Suicidal events tend to occur early in treatment.[22] Patients younger than 25 should be seen weekly for the first 4 weeks after initiation of treatment. Although less than ideal, patients can be monitored by phone if weekly appointments are impractical. Adherence should be monitored by use of a pill-count remainder, as nonadherence is associated with nonresponse,[46] and may also result in withdrawal symptoms that could precipitate suicidal behavior.

Strongly Consider Stopping the Antidepressant or Lowering the Dose in the Event of Adverse Effects

The occurrence of mania, agitation, akathisia, worsening of depression, severe anxiety, or new-onset suicidal ideation or behavior associated with initiation or a dose change should be taken seriously. Unless there are clear other reasons for these adverse events, the antidepressant dose should be lowered, or discontinued.

Rational Dosing

Start an antidepressant for the first week at half the initial target dose (ie, 10 mg fluoxetine). Starting at a high dose is associated with a higher risk of self-harm in adolescents and young adults.[43] Some studies find this association between a higher dose and higher risk of self-harm across the age span, rather than just in adolescence.[34,35] However, in patients who do not respond at a given dose may benefit from a dose increase.[17]

Identify and Target Risk Factors for Suicidal Events and Treatment Resistance

Clinicians should develop a safety plan for the adolescent and family, teach the patient distress tolerance (especially because depressive feelings are not likely to lift immediately after starting an antidepressant), and address sources of family discord.[47,48]

Try to Achieve as Rapid a Response in Treatment as Possible

There is some evidence that combination of medication and CBT will result in more rapid declines in suicidal ideation and depression.[49]

REFERENCES

1. Posner K, Oquendo MA, Gould M, et al. Columbia classification algorithm of suicide assessment (C-CASA): classification of suicidal events in the FDA's pediatric suicidal risk analysis of antidepressants. Am J Psychiatry 2007;164(7): 1035–43.

2. Hammad TA, Laughren T, Racoosin J. Suicidality in pediatric patients treated with antidepressant drugs. Arch Gen Psychiatry 2006;63(3):332–9.

3. Stone M, Laughren T, Jones ML, et al. Risk of suicidality in clinical trials of antidepressants in adults: analysis of proprietary data submitted to US Food and Drug Administration. BMJ 2009;339:b2880.

4. Bridge JA, Iyengar S, Salary CB, et al. Clinical response and risk for reported suicidal ideation and suicide attempts in pediatric antidepressant treatment: a meta-analysis of randomized controlled trials. JAMA 2007;297(15):1683–96.

5. Hetrick SE, McKenzie JE, Cox GR, et al. Newer generation antidepressants for depressive disorders in children and adolescents. Cochrane Database Syst Rev 2012;(11):CD004851.

6. Berk M, Dodd S. Are treatment emergent suicidality and decreased response to antidepressants in younger patients due to bipolar disorder being misdiagnosed as unipolar depression? Med Hypotheses 2005;65(1):39–43.

7. Martin A, Young C, Leckman JF, et al. Age effects on antidepressant-induced manic conversion. Arch Pediatr Adolesc Med 2004;158(8):773–80.

8. Offidani E, Fava GA, Tomba E, et al. Excessive mood elevation and behavioral activation with antidepressant treatment of juvenile depressive and anxiety disorders: a systematic review. Psychother Psychosom 2013;82(3):132–41.

9. Casey BJ, Jones RM, Levita L, et al. The storm and stress of adolescence: insights from human imaging and mouse genetics. Dev Psychobiol 2010;52(3): 225–35.

10. Tauscher J, Verhoeff NP, Christensen BK, et al. Serotonin 5-HT1A receptor binding potential declines with age as measured by [11C]WAY-100635 and PET. Neuropsychopharmacology 2001;24(5):522–30.

11. Moses-Kolko EL, Price JC, Shah N, et al. Age, sex, and reproductive hormone effects on brain serotonin-1A and serotonin-2A receptor binding in a healthy population. Neuropsychopharmacology 2011;36(13):2729–40.

12. Sullivan GM, Oquendo MA, Milak M, et al. Positron emission tomography quantification of serotonin(1A) receptor binding in suicide attempters with major depressive disorder. JAMA Psychiatry 2015;72(2):169–78.

13. Miller JM, Hesselgrave N, Ogden RT, et al. Brain serotonin 1A receptor binding as a predictor of treatment outcome in major depressive disorder. Biol Psychiatry 2013;74(10):760–7.

14. Oquendo MA, Russo SA, Underwood MD, et al. Higher postmortem prefrontal 5-HT2A receptor binding correlates with lifetime aggression in suicide. Biol Psychiatry 2006;59(3):235–43.
15. McGirr A, Renaud J, Bureau A, et al. Impulsive-aggressive behaviours and completed suicide across the life cycle: a predisposition for younger age of suicide. Psychol Med 2008;38(3):407–17.
16. Axelson DA, Perel JM, Birmaher B, et al. Sertraline pharmacokinetics and dynamics in adolescents. J Am Acad Child Adolesc Psychiatry 2002;41(9): 1037–44.
17. Sakolsky DJ, Perel JM, Emslie GJ, et al. Antidepressant exposure as a predictor of clinical outcomes in the Treatment of Resistant Depression in Adolescents (TORDIA) study. J Clin Psychopharmacol 2011;31(1):92–7.
18. Smith EG. Association between antidepressant half-life and the risk of suicidal ideation or behavior among children and adolescents: confirmatory analysis and research implications. J Affect Disord 2009;114(1–3):143–8.
19. Gibbons RD, Brown CH, Hur K, et al. Suicidal thoughts and behavior with antidepressant treatment: reanalysis of the randomized placebo-controlled studies of fluoxetine and venlafaxine. Arch Gen Psychiatry 2012;69(6):580–7.
20. Wichniak A, Wierzbicka A, Jernajczyk W. Sleep and antidepressant treatment. Curr Pharm Des 2012;18(36):5802–17.
21. Pigeon WR, Pinquart M, Conner K. Meta-analysis of sleep disturbance and suicidal thoughts and behaviors. J Clin Psychiatry 2012;73(9):e1160–1167.
22. Brent DA, Emslie GJ, Clarke GN, et al. Predictors of spontaneous and systematically assessed suicidal adverse events in the treatment of SSRI-resistant depression in adolescents (TORDIA) study. Am J Psychiatry 2009;166(4):418–26.
23. Mann JJ, Emslie G, Baldessarini RJ, et al. ACNP Task Force report on SSRIs and suicidal behavior in youth. Neuropsychopharmacology 2006;31(3):473–92.
24. Ludwig J, Marcotte DE. Anti-depressants, suicide, and drug regulation. J Policy Anal Manage 2005;24(2):249–72.
25. Gibbons RD, Hur K, Bhaumik DK, et al. The relationship between antidepressant medication use and rate of suicide. Arch Gen Psychiatry 2005;62(2):165–72.
26. Olfson M, Shaffer D, Marcus SC, et al. Relationship between antidepressant medication treatment and suicide in adolescents. Arch Gen Psychiatry 2003; 60(10):978–82.
27. Valuck RJ, Libby AM, Sills MR, et al. Antidepressant treatment and risk of suicide attempt by adolescents with major depressive disorder: a propensity-adjusted retrospective cohort study. CNS Drugs 2004;18(15):1119–32.
28. Tiihonen J, Lonnqvist J, Wahlbeck K, et al. Antidepressants and the risk of suicide, attempted suicide, and overall mortality in a nationwide cohort. Arch Gen Psychiatry 2006;63(12):1358–67.
29. Wijlaars LP, Nazareth I, Whitaker HJ, et al. Suicide-related events in young people following prescription of SSRIs and other antidepressants: a self-controlled case series analysis. BMJ Open 2013;3(9):e003247.
30. Simon GE, Savarino J, Operskalski B, et al. Suicide risk during antidepressant treatment. Am J Psychiatry 2006;163(1):41–7.
31. Gibbons RD, Coca Perraillon M, Hur K, et al. Antidepressant treatment and suicide attempts and self-inflicted injury in children and adolescents. Pharmacoepidemiol Drug Saf 2015;24(2):208–14.
32. Olfson M, Marcus SC, Shaffer D. Antidepressant drug therapy and suicide in severely depressed children and adults: a case-control study. Arch Gen Psychiatry 2006;63(8):865–72.

33. Leon AC, Marzuk PM, Tardiff K, et al. Paroxetine, other antidepressants, and youth suicide in New York City: 1993 through 1998. J Clin Psychiatry 2004; 65(7):915–8.

34. Courtet P, Lopez-Castroman J, Jaussent I, et al. Antidepressant dosage and suicidal ideation. JAMA Intern Med 2014;174(11):1863–5.

35. Coupland C, Hill T, Morriss R, et al. Antidepressant use and risk of suicide and attempted suicide or self-harm in people aged 20 to 64: cohort study using a primary care database. BMJ 2015;350:h517.

36. Gibbons RD, Brown CH, Hur K, et al. Early evidence on the effects of regulators' suicidality warnings on SSRI prescriptions and suicide in children and adolescents. Am J Psychiatry 2007;164(9):1356–63.

37. Libby AM, Orton HD, Valuck RJ. Persisting decline in depression treatment after FDA warnings. Arch Gen Psychiatry 2009;66(6):633–9.

38. Katz LY, Kozyrskyj AL, Prior HJ, et al. Effect of regulatory warnings on antidepressant prescription rates, use of health services and outcomes among children, adolescents and young adults. CMAJ 2008;178(8):1005–11.

39. Wheeler BW, Gunnell D, Metcalfe C, et al. The population impact on incidence of suicide and non-fatal self-harm of regulatory action against the use of selective serotonin reuptake inhibitors in under 18s in the United Kingdom: ecological study. BMJ 2008;336(7643):542–5.

40. Wilkinson P, Kelvin R, Roberts C, et al. Clinical and psychosocial predictors of suicide attempts and nonsuicidal self-injury in the adolescent depression antidepressants and psychotherapy trial (ADAPT). Am J Psychiatry 2011;168(5):495–501.

41. Asarnow JR, Porta G, Spirito A, et al. Suicide attempts and nonsuicidal self-injury in the treatment of resistant depression in adolescents: findings from the TORDIA study. J Am Acad Child Adolesc Psychiatry 2011;50(8):772–81.

42. March JS, Silva S, Petrycki S, et al. The treatment for adolescents with depression study (TADS): long-term effectiveness and safety outcomes. Arch Gen Psychiatry 2007;64(10):1132–43.

43. Miller M, Swanson SA, Azrael D, et al. Antidepressant dose, age, and the risk of deliberate self-harm. JAMA Intern Med 2014;174(6):899–909.

44. Schneeweiss S, Patrick AR, Solomon DH, et al. Variation in the risk of suicide attempts and completed suicides by antidepressant agent in adults: a propensity score-adjusted analysis of 9 years' data. Arch Gen Psychiatry 2010;67(5): 497–506.

45. American Academy of Child & Adolescent Psychiatry. Information for patients and their families. Available at: http://www.aacap.org/AACAP/Resources_for_Primary_Care/Information_for_Patients_and_Their_Families/Home.aspx?hkey=bce12396-b276-4fed-8430-ca8628eb1a2b. Accessed March 1, 2016.

46. Woldu H, Porta G, Goldstein T, et al. Pharmacokinetically and clinician-determined adherence to an antidepressant regimen and clinical outcome in the TORDIA trial. J Am Acad Child Adolesc Psychiatry 2011;50(5):490–8.

47. Maalouf FT, Atwi M, Brent DA. Treatment-resistant depression in adolescents: review and updates on clinical management. Depress Anxiety 2011;28(11):946–54.

48. Stanley B, Brown G, Brent DA, et al. Cognitive-behavioral therapy for suicide prevention (CBT-SP): treatment model, feasibility, and acceptability. J Am Acad Child Adolesc Psychiatry 2009;48(10):1005–13.

49. March J, Silva S, Petrycki S, et al. Fluoxetine, cognitive-behavioral therapy, and their combination for adolescents with depression: Treatment for Adolescents With Depression Study (TADS) randomized controlled trial. JAMA 2004;292(7): 807–20.

Adverse Effects of Electroconvulsive Therapy

Chittaranjan Andrade, MD[a],*, Shyam Sundar Arumugham, MD, DNB[b], Jagadisha Thirthalli, MD[b]

KEYWORDS

- Electroconvulsive therapy • Adverse effects • Complications • Cognition
- Risk factors

KEY POINTS

- Electroconvulsive therapy (ECT) is usually well tolerated; adverse effects (AEs) are commonly mild and self-limiting and can be managed symptomatically.
- Cardiovascular and cerebrovascular changes associated with ECT are usually uneventful in individuals without preexisting risk factors.
- In elderly individuals with preexisting risk factors, ECT can be administered safely under physiologic monitoring and with precautions to prevent and manage complications.
- Cognitive AEs are common but usually improve within a few weeks. Retrograde memory deficits may rarely persist.
- Modification of stimulus parameters and electrode placement help minimize cognitive AEs.

INTRODUCTION

The principal indications for electroconvulsive therapy (ECT) are depression, schizophrenia, and mania, and the commonest contexts of administration are when the patient is suicidal, catatonic, or medication-refractory. Use of ECT is limited, mainly because of its cognitive adverse effects (AEs). This article summarizes potential AEs of ECT.

ECT AEs mostly occur during or shortly after an ECT session and are attributable to the anesthesia, anticholinergic drug, muscle relaxant, electrical stimulus, or seizure. There are commonly more than 1 causative/contributing elements; these are not always easily identified.

Funding: No funding was involved in the preparation of this article.

Conflict of Interest: Nil related to this article.

[a] Department of Psychopharmacology, National Institute of Mental Health and Neurosciences, Hosur Road, Bangalore 560 029, India; [b] Department of Psychiatry, National Institute of Mental Health and Neurosciences, Hosur Road, Bangalore 560 029, India

* Corresponding author.

E-mail address: andradec@gmail.com

GENERAL ADVERSE EFFECTS THAT OCCUR AFTER ELECTROCONVULSIVE THERAPY

Patients may report dry mouth, nausea, headache, and myalgia after ECT. These AEs are usually mild and transient and so have been less systematically studied than cognitive AEs. Dry mouth is probably due to anticholinergic drugs in the premedication and is self-limiting.

Nausea

Post-ECT nausea may result from headache or anesthesia. Treating headache attenuates headache-related nausea. Anesthetic agents vary in nausea risk; propofol carries low risk[1] whereas ketamine carries higher risk.[2] Standard antiemetics can be prophylactically or therapeutically administered for post-ECT nausea.

Headache

Localized or diffuse post-ECT headache occurs in 26% to 85% of patients[3]; it should be differentiated from headache that often accompanies depression. Post-ECT headache is usually mild and self-limiting. It peaks within 2 hours of ECT and subsides within 24 hours.[4] It may rarely be severe and protracted, resembling vascular headache. Severe headache is commoner in youth and those with past history of headache.[4] Migraineurs may experience vascular headache after ECT.[5]

Conventional analgesics and triptans are effective for post-ECT headache.[6,7] Cryotherapy has also been found successful.[3,8] Analgesics administered pre-ECT may benefit patients with recurrent post-ECT headaches.[9]

Other Musculoskeletal Adverse Effects

Generalized myalgia of varying severity is common after an ECT session. The severity usually decreases after the first ECT.[4] The myalgia results from muscle fasciculations with depolarizing muscle relaxants, the convulsion, or both. Therefore, therapeutic and prophylactic measures, depending on the suspected etiology, include lower dosing with depolarizing muscle relaxants, use of nondepolarizing muscle relaxants, or better muscle relaxation and analgesics. Interestingly, some studies suggest that neither fasciculations nor convulsions correlate with myalgia severity.[4,10]

Compression fracture of thoracic vertebral bodies, fracture of long bones, dislocations, and muscle or ligament injuries are rare with modified ECT but may occur with unmodified treatments that are sometimes still used in some developing countries.[11] In this context, "unmodified" ECT refers to the administration of ECT without premedication; specifically, without the muscle relaxant.

If ECT technique is poor, biting of intraoral structures, loosening of teeth, and temporomandibular pain can occur.[12] Proper application of an appropriate bite block and firm mandibular closure during the seizure helps prevent such complications.

Other AEs occurring during and shortly after ECT are considered in the sections that follow.

ADVERSE EFFECTS DUE TO MUSCLE RELAXANTS

Seizure modification using succinylcholine or other agents may rarely result in AEs.

Prolonged Apnea

Succinylcholine apnea usually lasts a few minutes. It may prolong by a few more minutes in patients with high serum lithium levels, and to 30 minutes and beyond in patients genetically deficient in pseudocholinesterase, or after recent organophosphorus poisoning.[13–15] If apnea unexpectedly prolongs, respiratory support (under anesthesia) should continue until spontaneous breathing recommences; future muscle relaxation can be effected using nondepolarizing agents.[5]

Malignant Hyperthermia

Malignant hyperthermia is a rare, potentially life-threatening complication of inhalational anesthetics/succinylcholine that occurs in a few susceptible individuals. It is a hypermetabolic state involving skeletal muscles, presenting as muscle rigidity, fever, and acidosis, and must not be confused with neuroleptic malignant syndrome. Nondepolarizing muscle relaxants are preferred in individuals with past or family history of malignant hyperthermia.[16]

Hyperkalemia

Risk factors for succinylcholine-related hyperkalemia[17] are presented in **Box 1**.

Awareness Under Anesthesia

Administration of succinylcholine before the anesthesia has taken effect will result in the terrifying awareness of neuromuscular paralysis, detectable as sudden, unexplained, pre-ECT tachycardia. Memory of this awareness is usually obliterated by the administered ECT but may persist if the patient receives memory-sparing, right unilateral treatment. Good anesthesiological practice and monitoring of the depth of anesthesia using the bispectral index can prevent awareness under anesthesia.[18] The bispectral index is a proprietary algorithm that provides real-time analysis of the electroencephalogram (EEG) during anesthesia.

SEIZURE-RELATED ADVERSE EFFECTS
Prolonged Seizures

Prolonged seizures (>180 seconds), best detected using EEG, may occur in 1% to 2% of ECT-treated patients[19]; they increase the risk of post-ECT confusion and memory impairment.[20] Seizures longer than 120 seconds are best terminated using intravenous anesthesia, midazolam, or lorazepam. Propofol is then preferred anesthesia for future treatments.[21] Attention should be paid to risk factors[22] (**Box 2**).

Tardive Seizures

These are spontaneous seizures that very rarely occur during the post-ECT recovery period; risk factors are whatever lowers the seizure threshold, including drugs such as β-lactam antibiotics.[23] Tardive seizures include nonconvulsive and focal seizures (the latter may even involve the cerebral hemisphere contralateral to the side of electrode placement).[24] They are a sparsely reported complication with limited data on

---

Box 1
Risk factors for succinylcholine-related hyperkalemia

- Prolonged immobilization
- Burns
- Prolonged chemical denervation
- Severe infection
- Disuse atrophy
- Critical illness polyneuropathy/myopathy
- Upper or lower motor neuron lesions

Box 2
Risk factors for prolonged seizure

- Electrolyte disturbances
- Adolescence
- Drugs: lithium, theophylline, ciprofloxacin
- Anticonvulsant/alcohol/benzodiazepine withdrawal

---

prognosis and management. However, when ECT was resumed after removal of the suspected predisposing agent (eg, antibiotics) there were no further complications. ECT, by itself, raises the seizure threshold and so is not epileptogenic.

Status Epilepticus

Prolonged or tardive seizures may rarely persist as convulsive or nonconvulsive status epilepticus. Nonconvulsive status epilepticus manifests as unexplained abnormalities in mental state and behavior post-ECT, and must be differentiated from postictal confusion. EEG is diagnostic. Status epilepticus necessitates intravenous benzodiazepine administration.[22]

Todd Phenomena

Transient (commonly lasting only a few hours) neurologic deficits, such as aphasia, hemiparesis, or visual loss, may rarely arise immediately after ECT.[24–26] Absence of identifiable causes and spontaneous recovery suggest a Todd phenomenon (transient, postictal, focal neurologic deficits following seizures).[27] No intervention is necessary.

Postictal Confusional States

Postictal states characterized by anxiety, restlessness, and disorientation occur in 8% to 20% of patients receiving ECT.[28] These states are variously described as postictal agitation, confusion, or delirium. Prevention lies in paying attention to risk factors (**Box 3**). In patients at risk, prevention after ECT can be effected using parenteral

---

Box 3
Factors predisposing to postictal confusion

- Old age
- Comorbid brain disease (eg, Parkinson disease)
- Concurrent lithium use
- Pretreatment anxiety
- Inadequate anesthesia dose
- Use of ultrashort-acting anesthesia
- Inadequate muscle relaxation
- Bilateral electroconvulsive therapy (ECT)
- Sinusoidal wave ECT
- High-dose ECT
- Multiple ECT treatments during the same treatment session
- Daily ECT

---

anesthesia, benzodiazepines, or antipsychotics; treatment after onset can be effected using the same agents.[28,29]

CARDIAC ADVERSE EFFECTS

Cardiovascular complications, the commonest cause of morbidity and mortality with ECT,[30,31] have decreased with the institution of continuous heart rate, blood pressure, and electrocardiogram (ECG) monitoring, and improved anesthesiological technique. ECT can now be safely administered to most people, even those with preexisting cardiac disease.[32]

Parasympathetic activation, lasting for a few seconds and characterized by bradycardia, hypotension, and excessive oral secretions, occurs immediately after the ECT stimulus. It may result in transient asystole, premature ventricular contractions, and bradyarrhythmias. Anticholinergic premedication with atropine or glycopyrrolate helps prevent such complications. A subsequent sympathetic surge, lasting the duration of the seizure, results in tachycardia, hypertension, increased cardiac output, and increased myocardial oxygen demand; tachyarrhythmias and cardiac ischemia are possible complications. The sympathetic phase is reversed by another surge of parasympathetic activity. There may be a mild sympathetic discharge when the patient awakens.[30,32,33]

Cardiac autonomic changes may be attenuated or accentuated by preexisting cardiac disease, psychotropic medications, anesthesia, and ECT premedication. These factors need consideration when assessing cardiovascular risks with ECT.

The occurrence of any cardiac AE during ECT may be as high as 7.5% and 55.0% in patients without and with preexisting cardiac illness, respectively.[34] Events in healthy patients are generally transient and benign (eg, brief asystole, transitory arrhythmia); complications in patients with cardiac disease may include persistent arrhythmia or myocardial ischemia. A recent study of 450 consecutive patients (28% with cardiac illness) showed no significant cardiac complication in any patient receiving ECT[35]; in this study, high-risk patients were given prophylactic beta-blockers to attenuate the sympathetic surge during ECT.

Analysis of mortality in large sets of patients receiving ECT suggest that cardiovascular death shortly after ECT is very rare (approximately 4 per 100,000 sessions within 48 hours following ECT) and, in most cases, cannot be attributed to ECT, per se.[36,37]

Asystole

Transient asystole may occur due to stimulation of vagal nuclei after the electric stimulation. The risk is higher in youth without preexisting heart disease, and also after subconvulsive stimulation (eg, during stimulus dose titration) because of unimpeded parasympathetic activity. Succinylcholine and lithium may increase the risk of asystole. Such transient asystole has not been associated with serious consequences. Anticholinergic premedication is recommended if asystole complicated previous sessions,[38] but not as a routine because of a risk of tachycardia and cognitive AEs.

Raised Blood Pressure

Systolic blood pressure can reach 200 mm Hg because of the sympathetic surge during the seizure; the effect attenuates immediately after the seizure, rarely results in complications, and does not require treatment or prophylaxis unless the patient has a vulnerability (eg, ischemic heart disease, aneurysm anywhere), in which case intravenous beta-blockade during ECT attenuates risks.

Electrocardiogram Abnormalities

ECT may trigger transient ECG changes, such as ventricular ectopics, T-wave inversion, and ST depression[39]; these are usually benign and do not cause problems in healthy youth. However, such changes are more serious in patients with cardiac illness. Suspected myocardial ischemia should be evaluated with troponin levels (creatine phosphokinase levels may be falsely elevated by the convulsion). Atropine and beta-blockers can be used for treatment-emergent bradyarrhythmias and tachyarrhythmias, respectively.

Myocardial Infarction

Myocardial infarction (MI)[40] and cardiac rupture[41] may rarely occur in patients with multiple cardiac risk factors. Patients with recent MI may suffer reinfarction, and so ECT is best avoided within 3 months of MI.[30] However, ECT has been safely administered after recent MI, even as early as 10 days after MI, with efficient cardiac management.[42] Treatment decisions in such situations are made case-by-case after cardiology consultation and stabilization of cardiac status. Intravenous labetalol/esmolol during ECT will reduce myocardial demands[43]; propofol anesthesia may be associated with less adverse hemodynamic change.

Cardiomyopathy

ECT may cause transient, clinically insignificant, wall motion abnormalities, detectable using echocardiography. Transient, reversible, sympathetic surge stress-induced Takotsubo cardiomyopathy may rarely follow ECT[22,44]; resumption of ECT, if required, should be undertaken with concomitant use of beta-blockers such as esmolol or labetolol.[45,46]

Factors that moderate cardiac AEs are listed in **Box 4**.

RESPIRATORY ADVERSE EFFECTS

Aspiration leading to pneumonitis,[47,48] neurogenic pulmonary edema,[49,50] and pulmonary embolism[51] may rarely complicate ECT.

NEUROLOGIC ADVERSE EFFECTS

Cerebral blood flow may treble during ECT,[30] catering to the increased oxygen demand during the seizure. An increased vascular permeability may lead to temporary functional breakdown in the blood brain barrier.[52] These changes may increase intracranial tension and sometimes cause transient, benign brain edema; however, complications may arise in patients with preexisting central nervous system (CNS) lesions.

Ischemic stroke is rare after ECT,[53,54] and whether ECT is causal is debatable. ECT has been used safely in post-(ischemic) stroke depression. After hemorrhagic stroke, aggressive beta-blockade is necessary to reduce the ECT-induced sympathetic surge and the risk of rebleed. After ischemic stroke, aggressive antihypertensive measures should be avoided due to risk of hypotensive morbidity.[30]

Despite the theoretic risk of bleeding, many patients with treated and untreated aneurysm and arteriovenous malformation have safely received ECT moderated by control of the hypertensive surge.[55,56]

Electroconvulsive Therapy and Brain Damage

Extensive research in animal models and humans, using neurohistological, brain imaging, and other investigational methods, has failed to find evidence of structural

---

Box 4
Factors that moderate cardiac adverse effects of ECT

Preexisting cardiac disease

- Recent myocardial infarction and uncontrolled hypertension carry a high risk for adverse cardiovascular outcomes. The decision for ECT should be made after evaluating the risk of not treating the psychiatric condition (eg, suicide) vis-à-vis the risk associated with ECT.

- Patients with asymptomatic mild arrhythmias, such as first-degree heart block or bundle branch block, can be safely treated with ECT.

- Severe heart block and ventricular arrhythmias are high-risk conditions for ECT.

- Atrial fibrillation may convert to normal sinus rhythm during ECT, increasing the risk of embolism. Prophylactic anticoagulation may be helpful.

Electrode placement

- Bifrontal ECT is associated with less vagal stimulation than bitemporal ECT.

Anesthetic agents

- Propofol is associated with less hemodynamic response and may be preferable in patients with cardiac disease. Methohexital is also considered to carry a lower risk of cardiac complications. Etomidate is preferred in congestive cardiac failure as it is less likely to cause hypotension. Ketamine accentuates the hemodynamic response. Thiopentone may cause bradycardia and ventricular premature contractions.

Subconvulsive stimulation

- This increases the risk of cardiac asystole.

Age

- Younger age is associated with asystole. Older age increases risks of other complications because of cardiac and other comorbidity.

Psychotropic drugs

- Drugs with anticholinergic effects may increase tachycardia; drugs that block alpha-1 adrenoceptors may predispose to bradyarrhythmias and hypotension

Data from Refs.[30,31,33,38,91]

---

brain damage with ECT[57]; rather, ECT has emerged as a potent inducer of neuroplasticity.[58] The available data suggest that the stimulus parameters during ECT and the duration of the ECT seizure are well below the threshold associated with risk for neuronal damage.

COGNITIVE IMPAIRMENT

Memory and nonmemory cognitive AEs (CogAEs) are a vexing consequence of ECT[59]; the extent of their persistence is much debated,[60] and their identification and measurement are confounded by many factors (**Box 5**). ECT-related CogAEs may be acute, subacute, and persistent effects, as explained in **Box 6**.

Certain cognitive domains can improve with ECT as the underlying illness remits.[61] As an example, cognitive deficits associated with depression exemplify impaired acquisition of information, whereas those arising from ECT exemplify impaired retention. These 2 categories of deficits are described by different test items and dissociate across the course of ECT: as the former decrease, the latter increase.[62]

> **Box 5**
> **Factors confounding identification and evaluation of cognitive adverse events with ECT**
>
> - The nature and severity of the disorder for which ECT is administered. All psychiatric disorders are associated with varying degrees of cognitive impairment, and the greater the severity of the disorder, the greater the impairment.
>
> - The nature and dose of concurrent psychotropic medication. Most psychotropic drugs dose-dependently impair cognitive processes.
>
> - The nature and dose of ECT premedication. Anesthesia and anticholinergic drugs both impair cognition, the former more measurably than the latter.
>
> - The degree of residual psychiatric impairment after ECT. If illness persists, its cognitive effects will also persist.

Nonmemory Cognitive Deficits

Studies on non-memory cognitive functioning show worsening, improvement or no change after ECT,[63] perhaps because of clinical confounds (see **Box 5**). A meta-analysis of studies in ECT-treated depression[61] found that, relative to a pre-ECT baseline status, medium to large short-term (up to 3 days post-ECT) deficits existed in episodic memory and executive functioning, and small deficits existed in processing speed, spatial problem-solving, and global cognition. Attention and working memory did not differ from baseline. Reassuringly, all deficits attenuated across 15 days post-ECT, and improvements, beyond baseline, were identified in many domains. There was no evidence for deficit in intellectual ability after ECT. It appears that ECT may not cause lasting deficits in various non-memory cognitive domains; improvements recorded may be secondary to improvement in the underlying illness.

MEMORY LOSS

ECT has no effects on implicit learning and memory, such as skill learning and perceptual priming.[64] Most studies have focused on the effect of ECT on declarative/explicit memory. ECT has different effects on verbal and nonverbal, episodic and semantic, explicit memory; these are best described under anterograde and retrograde amnesia, as they are governed by different neurobiological substrates.

> **Box 6**
> **Acute, subacute, and chronic cognitive adverse effects (CogAEs) of ECT**
>
> - Acute CogAEs occur immediately after ECT. They manifest as deficits in attention and immediate memory; sometimes, even orientation may be impaired. They present as postictal confusion or delirium in severe forms. Prolonged postictal disorientation predicts greater subacute retrograde amnesia.
>
> - Acute CogAEs are transient and self-limiting; recovery usually occurs within an hour. Postictal confusion or delirium will require medical termination.
>
> - Subacute CogAEs include anterograde and retrograde amnesia, and nonmemory cognitive deficits. These attenuate weeks to months after ECT.
>
> - Chronic CogAEs persist for months or longer, and comprise retrograde amnestic deficits.
>
> - Whether ECT causes permanent CogAEs is hotly debated.

Anterograde Amnesia

Anterograde amnesia refers to impairment of new learning; that is, impaired recall of material learned or events occurring after the commencement of the ECT course. Clinically significant anterograde memory deficits are usually evident during the ECT course. Anterograde amnestic deficits implicate memory retention (delayed recall) more than memory acquisition (immediate recall)[61,63]; and acquisition recovers earlier than retention.[62] Examples and characteristics of anterograde amnesia are presented in **Boxes 7** and **8**, respectively.

Retrograde (Including Autobiographical) Amnesia

Retrograde amnesia refers to forgetting of material learned or events occurring before ECT. Retrograde amnesia is arguably the most debated and treatment-limiting adverse effect of ECT. This is because (episodic) memories are strongly tied to a sense of identity,[65] and so loss of personal (autobiographical) memories is perceived as damaging. Examples and characteristics of retrograde amnesia are presented in **Boxes 8** and **9**, respectively. Both episodic and semantic retrograde amnesia occur with ECT; the extent of amnesia is variable, and the permanence of loss is debated.[59]

   The assessment of autobiographical memory (**Box 10**) across the life span presents difficulties. Many standardized tests exist for the assessment of different aspects of autobiographic memory; these may yield inconsistent results. Some studies show that autobiographical memory loss may persist up to 3 years after ECT.[66] It has been suggested that approximately 1 in 200 patients may experience severe and/or long-lasting memory deficits with ECT.[67] This, coupled with personal accounts citing permanent autobiographical memory loss after ECT,[68] have made autobiographical memory loss the most reviled adverse effect of ECT.

Subjective Memory Loss

Patients may report subjective memory loss with ECT months or even years after the ECT course; however, objective neuropsychological impairment is rarely identifiable in these patients. Assessments of subjective memory loss using, for example, the Squire Subjective Memory Questionnaire, correlate poorly with objective cognitive testing but more strongly with severity of depression.[69] Some investigators suggest that some of the subjective memory loss after ECT may be manifestations of somatoform disorder.[70] Possible explanations for wholly subjective memory complaints are presented in **Box 11**.

Moderators of Electroconvulsive Therapy–Induced Amnesia

Factors that predispose to increased ECT-induced amnesia are presented in **Box 12**. A modification of treatment-related factors can help reduce memory loss with ECT.[71] For example, in patients with increased predisposition for cognitive AEs, lower dose of anesthesia, right unilateral or bifrontal electrode placement, ultrabrief-pulse ECT,

---

Box 7
Examples of anterograde amnesia

- Test example: There is impaired performance on neuropsychological tasks of learning and memory during and immediately after the ECT course.

- Real-life example: The patient is hazy about details of events that occur during and shortly after the ECT course; this can be elicited through questioning not only during the ECT course but in later weeks, as well.

> **Box 8**
> **Characteristics of ECT-induced amnesia**
>
> - Anterograde and retrograde amnesia both cumulate across the ECT course; that is, they increase with the number of ECTs administered.
> - Anterograde and retrograde amnesia both exhibit a temporal gradient; that is, the amnesia is most severe for events close to the ECT course and diminishes in intensity with increasing temporal distance from the ECT course.
> - Anterograde amnesia attenuates days to weeks after ECT, and return of learning abilities to the pre-ECT baseline (or better, especially if the illness has remitted) is substantially complete within a month.
> - Retrograde amnesia slowly attenuates weeks to months after ECT. However, many patients experience long-lasting, patchy memory deficits, particularly for events during and around the ECT course. Some patients may have difficulty in recalling events that occurred years before the treatment.
> - Nonautobiographical memories are emotionally less salient and less rehearsed, and are therefore more sensitive than autobiographical memories to the amnesiogenic effects of ECT.
> - Permanent anterograde amnesia does not occur, but permanent retrograde autobiographical and nonautobiographical amnesia of varying severity has been anecdotally described; the etiologic role of ECT in this regard is debated.

lower ECT stimulus charge, and so forth, may reduce CogAEs. These strategies should be implemented after analyzing the risk/benefit ratio of the modifications.

Monitoring Cognitive Adverse Effects

Cognition should be assessed at baseline, during, and at the end of the ECT course in all patients receiving ECT. Global measures, such as the Mini Mental State Examination (MMSE),[72] are probably insensitive to ECT CogAEs. However, lower baseline MMSE score (indicating poor baseline cognitive functioning) is associated with more severe retrograde memory deficits post-ECT.[73,74] Longer time to reorientation following ECT is another predictor of retrograde memory deficits.[73,74] Batteries for rapid cognitive assessment of ECT-specific deficits (eg, anterograde memory, autobiographic memory) are recommended for monitoring of cognitive AEs.[75,76]

Pharmacologic Prevention of Electroconvulsive Therapy–Induced Amnesia

Many drugs have been studied for the reduction of cognitive deficits with ECT; these drugs range from nootropic agents to thyroid hormones and even donepezil. Although positive findings have been obtained in animal research and in a few clinical trials, no drug has been shown to consistently benefit patients treated with ECT.[77] At present,

> **Box 9**
> **Examples of retrograde amnesia**
>
> - Test example: There is impaired recall of details of life incidents that the patient described to the physician (as part of the autobiographical memory test baseline assessment) before the start of the ECT course.
> - Real-life example: The patient is hazy about details related to his admission to the hospital for the administration of ECT.

Box 10
Examples of autobiographical amnesia

- Forgetting of details related to school, college, family, and leisure life (episodic memories).
- Forgetting of names, dates, telephone numbers, and addresses (semantic memories).

---

therefore, no medication can be recommended to attenuate ECT-related cognitive impairment.

EFFECTS OF ELECTROCONVULSIVE THERAPY ON PREGNANCY

A recent review of case reports of ECT use in pregnancy indicates a high risk of complications (29.1%) and a fetal mortality rate of 7.1%.[78] This review is in contrast with others that report far lower risks.[79–81] None of these reviews could accurately estimate the incidence of adverse outcomes, nor could the adverse events be definitively attributable to ECT. Adverse outcomes (**Box 13**) in pregnant women who have received ECT may be due to spontaneous events, underlying psychiatric conditions, use of psychotropic medications, and ECT procedures. **Box 14** lists precautions for ECT during pregnancy.

MISCELLANEOUS ADVERSE EFFECTS

An organic affective syndrome, transient treatment-emergent mania, and manic switch have variously been described to develop in 3% to 10% of patients with depression who receive ECT.[82] Transient hypomania followed by return into depression may rarely arise midway during an ECT-treated depressive episode.[83,84] Should a patient relapse into depression after rapid and spontaneous resolution of such hypomania, it is probably best to resume ECT with an intent to treat the patient to euthymia.

Extremely rare AEs include urinary bladder rupture, gastric rupture, vitreous detachment, and bleeding at various sites.[11,85–87]

COMBINING ELECTROCONVULSIVE THERAPY WITH PSYCHOTROPIC DRUGS

Patients receiving ECT are often prescribed psychotropic medications for prevention of relapse after completion of the course of ECT. Careful attention is required with regard to AEs when ECT is combined with certain psychotropic medications. There may be risk of prolonged seizures and delirium when ECT is administered to patients on lithium, especially in people with advanced age, brain lesions, and high serum lithium levels.[5,15] Clozapine can be safely combined with ECT with some attention given to

---

Box 11
Possible causes of persistent subjective memory impairment or loss with ECT

- The complaints about post-ECT memory impairment or loss may be genuine and may truly be due to ECT but are too mild to be detected by conventional neuropsychological tests.
- The complaints may represent a true decline from baseline but result from other factors such as increasing age or the psychiatric illness, itself.
- There is no true decline from baseline and the subjective memory impairment or loss comprise misattributions of normal forgetfulness to the effects of ECT.

Box 12
Risk factors for ECT-induced amnesia

Patient related

- Old age
- Diminished cognitive reserve
- Existing brain disease

Treatment related

- Concomitant psychotropic agents; for example, lithium
- Higher anesthesia dose and, possibly, use of anticholinergics in the premedication
- Bilateral ECT, especially bitemporal electrode placement
- Sinusoidal wave ECT
- High-dose ECT
- Greater frequency of ECT
- Greater number of ECT treatments

---

possible tachycardia, delirium, and prolonged seizures.[88] There are no specific concerns while combining other antipsychotics with ECT, except that it may be best to avoid drugs that have alpha adrenergic blocking properties. Most antidepressants can be safely prescribed, but there are theoretic concerns regarding anticholinergic AEs and cardiotoxicity when ECT is combined with high doses of tricyclic antidepressants.[5] Beta-blockers, such as propranolol, may increase the risk of bradycardia and asystole if there is a subconvulsive stimulation. Benzodiazepines and anticonvulsants increase seizure threshold and hence their dosing may have to be modified during the course of ECT.

MORTALITY RISK WITH ELECTROCONVULSIVE THERAPY

Deaths directly or plausibly attributed to the electrical stimulus, seizure, or anesthesia during ECT are estimated to be approximately 2 to 10 per 100,000 treatments.[36] Naturalistic comparative studies suggest that mortality among patients treated with ECT is actually lower than those receiving alternate treatments.[89,90] Cardiac and respiratory events are the most common causes of mortality related to ECT procedures; the deaths are commonly attributable to preexisting medical illness and anesthesia-related complications.[36,37]

Box 13
Pregnancy complications reported during ECT

Maternal complications

- Gastric reflux, uterine contractions, vaginal bleeding, abruptio placentae, abortion/premature labor, cesarean delivery[a]

Fetal complications

- Fetal bradycardia, neonatal death,[a] congenital anomalies[a]

    [a] May not be related to ECT.

Box 14
Procedures and precautions for ECT during pregnancy

- Administer ECT in an in-patient setting with facilities available to manage complications
- Obtain informed consent after explaining possible fetal and maternal complications
- Involve the obstetrician in planning treatment
- Stop anticholinergic drugs, if possible
- Monitor fetal heart rate during ECT
- Elevate right hip, especially during the third trimester
- Ensure adequate hydration
- Avoid excessive hyperventilation
- Consider prophylactic administration of antacid to reduce consequences of reflux
- Administer tocolytic treatment, if required

IMPLICATIONS FOR INFORMED CONSENT

It is important that treating psychiatrists educate patients and caregivers regarding potential AEs while recommending ECT. Common adverse events, including headache, nausea, myalgia, and transient cognitive deficits, should be differentiated from uncommon but potentially serious adverse events, including anesthetic and cardiovascular complications. The possibility of long-term patchy retrograde amnesia, although debated, should be explained. In patients with higher risk for complications, including those with preexisting cardiac illness, CNS lesions, and so forth, the risk-benefit analysis should be discussed in detail.

SUMMARY

Nearly 80 years after its introduction and despite the current availability of scores of antidepressant, antipsychotic, mood stabilizer, and other drugs, ECT remains an important treatment in psychiatry. Proper pre-ECT evaluation of risk, adoption of appropriate risk mitigation measures, good anesthesia technique, seizure modification, brief-pulse and possibly ultrabrief-pulse stimulation, unilateral and possibly bifrontal electrode placement, stimulus dose titration, ECG and EEG monitoring during ECT, cognitive monitoring during the ECT course, and other strategies will all go a long way toward attenuating AEs with the treatment.

REFERENCES

1. Shah PJ, Dubey KP, Watti C, et al. Effectiveness of thiopentone, propofol and midazolam as an ideal intravenous anaesthetic agent for modified electroconvulsive therapy: a comparative study. Indian J Anaesth 2010;54(4):296–301.
2. Salehi B, Mohammadbeigi A, Kamali AR, et al. Impact comparison of ketamine and sodium thiopental on anesthesia during electroconvulsive therapy in major depression patients with drug-resistant; a double-blind randomized clinical trial. Ann Card Anaesth 2015;18(4):486–90.
3. Drew BI, King ML, Callahan L. Cryotherapy for treatment of ECT-induced headache. J Psychosoc Nurs Ment Health Serv 2005;43(4):32–9.
4. Dinwiddie SH, Huo D, Gottlieb O. The course of myalgia and headache after electroconvulsive therapy. J ECT 2010;26(2):116–20.

5. American Psychiatric Association. The practice of electroconvulsive therapy-recommendations for treatment, training, and privileging (A Task Force Report of the American Psychiatric Association). 2nd edition. Washington, DC: American Psychiatric Press; 2001.
6. Markowitz JS, Kellner CH, DeVane CL, et al. Intranasal sumatriptan in post-ECT headache: results of an open-label trial. J ECT 2001;17(4):280–3.
7. Kertesz DP, Trabekin O, Vanetik MS. Headache treatment after electroconvulsive treatment: a single-blinded trial comparator between eletriptan and paracetamol. J ECT 2015;31(2):105–9.
8. Kramer BA, Kadar AG, Clark K. Use of the neuro-wrap system for severe post-electroconvulsive therapy headaches. J ECT 2008;24(2):152–5.
9. Leung M, Hollander Y, Brown GR. Pretreatment with ibuprofen to prevent electroconvulsive therapy-induced headache. J Clin Psychiatry 2003;64(5):551–3.
10. Rasmussen KG, Petersen KN, Sticka JL, et al. Correlates of myalgia in electroconvulsive therapy. J ECT 2008;24(1):84–7.
11. Andrade C, Shah N, Tharyan P, et al. Position statement and guidelines on unmodified electroconvulsive therapy. Indian J Psychiatry 2012;54(2):119–33.
12. Woo S-W, Do S-H. Tongue laceration during electroconvulsive therapy. Korean J Anesthesiol 2012;62(1):101–2.
13. Moudi S, Alijanpour E, Manouchehri A-A, et al. A case report of prolonged apnea during ECT in a patient with suicidal attempt by organophosphorus poison. Iran J Psychiatry Behav Sci 2012;6(1):68–71.
14. Waghmare A, Kumar CN, Thirthalli J. Suxamethonium induced prolonged apnea in a patient receiving electroconvulsive therapy. Gen Hosp Psychiatry 2010;32(4):447.e1–2.
15. Thirthalli J, Harish T, Gangadhar BN. A prospective comparative study of interaction between lithium and modified electroconvulsive therapy. World J Biol Psychiatry 2011;12(2):149–55.
16. Yacoub OF, Morrow DH. Malignant hyperthermia and ECT. Am J Psychiatry 1986;143(8):1027–9.
17. Martyn JAJ, Richtsfeld M. Succinylcholine-induced hyperkalemia in acquired pathologic states: etiologic factors and molecular mechanisms. Anesthesiology 2006;104(1):158–69.
18. Andrade C, Thirthalli J, Gangadhar BN. Unilateral nondominant electrode placement as a risk factor for recall of awareness under anesthesia during electroconvulsive therapy. J ECT 2007;23(3):201–3.
19. Whittaker R, Scott A, Gardner M. The prevalence of prolonged cerebral seizures at the first treatment in a course of electroconvulsive therapy. J ECT 2007;23(1):11–3.
20. Whitehouse AM, Scott AIF. Monitoring seizure activity. The ECT handbook: the third report of the Royal College of Psychiatrists' Special Committee of ECT. 2nd edition. London: The Royal College of Psychiatrists; 2005. p. 159–69.
21. Aloysi AS, Bryson EO, Kellner CH. Management of prolonged seizures during electroconvulsive therapy. Indian J Psychol Med 2014;36(2):220–1.
22. Cristancho MA, Alici Y, Augoustides JG, et al. Uncommon but serious complications associated with electroconvulsive therapy: recognition and management for the clinician. Curr Psychiatry Rep 2008;10(6):474–80.
23. Saito T, Nakamura M, Watari M, et al. Tardive seizure and antibiotics: case reports and review of the literature. J ECT 2008;24(4):275–6.
24. Felkel WC, Wagner G, Kimball J, et al. Tardive seizure with postictal aphasia: a case report. J ECT 2012;28(3):180–2.

25. Kurani AP, Kellner CH, Turbin RE, et al. Transient visual loss after right unilateral ECT. J ECT 2005;21(3):186–7.
26. Liff JM, Bryson EO, Maloutas E, et al. Transient hemiparesis (Todd's paralysis) after electroconvulsive therapy (ECT) in a patient with major depressive disorder. J ECT 2013;29(3):247–8.
27. Todd RB. The Lumleian Lectures for 1849. On the pathology and treatment of convulsive diseases. Epilepsia 2005;46(7):995–1009.
28. Tzabazis A, Schmitt HJ, Ihmsen H, et al. Postictal agitation after electroconvulsive therapy: incidence, severity, and propofol as a treatment option. J ECT 2013; 29(3):189–95.
29. Bryson EO, Briggs MC, Pasculli RM, et al. Treatment-resistant postictal agitation after electroconvulsive therapy (ECT) controlled with dexmedetomidine. J ECT 2013;29(2):e18.
30. Rabheru K. The use of electroconvulsive therapy in special patient populations. Can J Psychiatry 2001;46(8):710–9.
31. Rasmussen KG, Rummans TA, Richardson JW. Electroconvulsive therapy in the medically ill. Psychiatr Clin North Am 2002;25(1):177–93.
32. Tess AV, Smetana GW. Medical evaluation of patients undergoing electroconvulsive therapy: current concepts. N Engl J Med 2009;360(14):1437–44.
33. Christopher EJ. Electroconvulsive therapy in the medically ill. Curr Psychiatry Rep 2003;5(3):225–30.
34. Zielinski RJ, Roose SP, Devanand DP, et al. Cardiovascular complications of ECT in depressed patients with cardiac disease. Am J Psychiatry 1993;150(6): 904–9.
35. Bryson EO, Popeo D, Briggs M, et al. Electroconvulsive therapy (ECT) in patients with cardiac disease: hemodynamic changes. J ECT 2013;29(1):76–7.
36. Shiwach RS, Reid WH, Carmody TJ. An analysis of reported deaths following electroconvulsive therapy in Texas, 1993-1998. Psychiatr Serv 2001;52(8): 1095–7.
37. Østergaard SD, Bolwig TG, Petrides G. No causal association between electroconvulsive therapy and death: a summary of a report from the Danish Health and Medicines Authority covering 99,728 treatments. J ECT 2014;30(4):263–4.
38. Roche NC, Raynaud L, Bompaire F, et al. Per stimulus asystole during electroconvulsive therapy: clinical case and critical literature review. Encephale 2016;42(1): 59–66 [in French].
39. Narasimhan S. Electroconvulsive therapy and electrocardiograph changes. J Postgrad Med 2008;54(3):228.
40. López-Gómez D, Sánchez-Corral MA, Cobo JV, et al. Myocardial infarction after electroconvulsive therapy. Rev Esp Cardiol 1999;52(7):536 [in Spanish].
41. Ali PB, Tidmarsh MD. Cardiac rupture during electroconvulsive therapy. Anaesthesia 1997;52(9):884–6.
42. Magid M, Lapid MI, Sampson SM, et al. Use of electroconvulsive therapy in a patient 10 days after myocardial infarction. J ECT 2005;21(3):182–5.
43. Boere E, Birkenhäger TK, Groenland THN, et al. Beta-blocking agents during electroconvulsive therapy: a review. Br J Anaesth 2014;113(1):43–51.
44. Narayanan A, Russell MD, Sundararaman S, et al. Takotsubo cardiomyopathy following electroconvulsive therapy: an increasingly recognised phenomenon. BMJ Case Rep 2014;2014. http://dx.doi.org/10.1136/bcr-2014-206816.
45. Celano CM, Torri A, Seiner S. Takotsubo cardiomyopathy after electroconvulsive therapy: a case report and review. J ECT 2011;27(3):221–3.

46. de Wolf MM, Olde Bijvank EGM. Takotsubo cardiomyopathy as a complication of electroconvulsive therapy. Tijdschr Psychiatr 2015;57(5):361–6 [in Dutch].

47. Kurnutala LN, Kamath S, Koyfman S, et al. Aspiration during electroconvulsive therapy under general anesthesia. J ECT 2013;29(4):e68.

48. Zibrak JD, Jensen WA, Bloomingdale K. Aspiration pneumonitis following electroconvulsive therapy in patients with gastroparesis. Biol Psychiatry 1988; 24(7):812–4.

49. Takahashi T, Kinoshita K, Fuke T, et al. Acute neurogenic pulmonary edema following electroconvulsive therapy: a case report. Gen Hosp Psychiatry 2012; 34(6):703.e9–11.

50. Manne JR, Kasirye Y, Epperla N, et al. Non-cardiogenic pulmonary edema complicating electroconvulsive therapy: short review of the pathophysiology and diagnostic approach. Clin Med Res 2012;10(3):131–6.

51. Mamah D, Lammle M, Isenberg KE. Pulmonary embolism after ECT. J ECT 2005; 21(1):39–40.

52. Andrade C, Bolwig TG. Electroconvulsive therapy, hypertensive surge, blood-brain barrier breach, and amnesia: exploring the evidence for a connection. J ECT 2014;30(2):160–4.

53. Lee K. Acute embolic stroke after electroconvulsive therapy. J ECT 2006;22(1):67–9.

54. Bruce BB, Henry ME, Greer DM. Ischemic stroke after electroconvulsive therapy. J ECT 2006;22(2):150–2.

55. van Herck E, Sienaert P, Hagon A. Electroconvulsive therapy for patients with intracranial aneurysms: a case study and literature review. Tijdschr Psychiatr 2009;51(1):43–51 [in Dutch].

56. Wilkinson ST, Helgeson L, Ostroff RB. Electroconvulsive therapy and cerebral aneurysms. J ECT 2014;30(4):47–9.

57. Devanand DP, Dwork AJ, Hutchinson ER, et al. Does ECT alter brain structure? Am J Psychiatry 1994;151(7):957–70.

58. Bouckaert F, Sienaert P, Obbels J, et al. ECT: its brain enabling effects: a review of electroconvulsive therapy-induced structural brain plasticity. J ECT 2014;30(2): 143–51.

59. Sackeim HA. Memory and ECT: from polarization to reconciliation. J ECT 2000; 16(2):87–96.

60. Abrams R. Does bilateral ECT cause persistent cognitive impairment? J ECT 2007;23(2):61–2.

61. Semkovska M, McLoughlin DM. Objective cognitive performance associated with electroconvulsive therapy for depression: a systematic review and meta-analysis. Biol Psychiatry 2010;68(6):568–77.

62. Steif BL, Sackeim HA, Portnoy S, et al. Effects of depression and ECT on antero-grade memory. Biol Psychiatry 1986;21(10):921–30.

63. Ingram A, Saling MM, Schweitzer I. Cognitive side effects of brief pulse electro-convulsive therapy: a review. J ECT 2008;24(1):3–9.

64. Vakil E, Grunhaus L, Nagar I, et al. The effect of electroconvulsive therapy (ECT) on implicit memory: skill learning and perceptual priming in patients with major depression. Neuropsychologia 2000;38(10):1405–14.

65. King MJ, MacDougall AG, Ferris SM, et al. A review of factors that moderate auto-biographical memory performance in patients with major depressive disorder. J Clin Exp Neuropsychol 2010;32(10):1122–44.

66. Squire LR, Slater PC. Electroconvulsive therapy and complaints of memory dysfunction: a prospective three-year follow-up study. Br J Psychiatry 1983; 142:1–8.

67. Fink M. Convulsive therapy: theory and practice. New York: Raven Press; 1979.

68. Donahue AB. Electroconvulsive therapy and memory loss: a personal journey. J ECT 2000;16(2):133–43.

69. Fraser LM, O'Carroll RE, Ebmeier KP. The effect of electroconvulsive therapy on autobiographical memory: a systematic review. J ECT 2008;24(1):10–7.

70. Fink M. Complaints of loss of personal memories after electroconvulsive therapy: evidence of a somatoform disorder? Psychosomatics 2007;48(4):290–3.

71. McClintock SM, Choi J, Deng Z-D, et al. Multifactorial determinants of the neurocognitive effects of electroconvulsive therapy. J ECT 2014;30(2):165–76.

72. Folstein MF, Folstein SE, McHugh PR. Mini-mental state. J Psychiatr Res 1975; 12(3):189–98.

73. Sobin C, Sackeim HA, Prudic J, et al. Predictors of retrograde amnesia following ECT. Am J Psychiatry 1995;152(7):995–1001.

74. Martin DM, Gálvez V, Loo CK. Predicting retrograde autobiographical memory changes following electroconvulsive therapy: relationships between individual, treatment, and early clinical factors. Int J Neuropsychopharmacol 2015. http://dx.doi.org/10.1093/ijnp/pyv067.

75. Viswanath B, Harihara SN, Nahar A, et al. Battery for ECT related cognitive deficits (B4ECT-ReCoDe): development and validation. Asian J Psychiatr 2013;6(3): 243–8.

76. Martin DM, Katalinic N, Ingram A, et al. A new early cognitive screening measure to detect cognitive side-effects of electroconvulsive therapy? J Psychiatr Res 2013;47(12):1967–74.

77. Pigot M, Andrade C, Loo C. Pharmacological attenuation of electroconvulsive therapy–induced cognitive deficits: theoretical background and clinical findings. J ECT 2008;24(1):57–67.

78. Leiknes KA, Cooke MJ, Jarosch-von Schweder L, et al. Electroconvulsive therapy during pregnancy: a systematic review of case studies. Arch Womens Ment Health 2015;18(1):1–39.

79. Anderson EL, Reti IM. ECT in pregnancy: a review of the literature from 1941 to 2007. Psychosom Med 2009;71(2):235–42.

80. Miller LJ. Use of electroconvulsive therapy during pregnancy. Hosp Community Psychiatry 1994;45(5):444–50.

81. Pompili M, Dominici G, Giordano G, et al. Electroconvulsive treatment during pregnancy: a systematic review. Expert Rev Neurother 2014;14(12):1377–90.

82. Devanand DP, Sackeim HA, Decina P, et al. The development of mania and organic euphoria during ECT. J Clin Psychiatry 1988;49(2):69–71.

83. Andrade C, Gangadhar BN, Swaminath G, et al. Mania as a side effect of electroconvulsive therapy. Convuls Ther 1988;4(1):81–3.

84. Andrade C, Gangadhar BN, Channabasavanna SM. Further characterization of mania as a side effect of ECT. Convuls Ther 1990;6(4):318–9.

85. Irving AD, Drayson AM. Bladder rupture during ECT. Br J Psychiatry J Ment Sci 1984;144:670.

86. van Schaik AM, Klumpers UMH, de Gast HM, et al. Gastric rupture after electroconvulsive therapy. J ECT 2006;22(2):153–4.

87. Martínez-Amorós E, Real Barrero E, Fuste Fusares C, et al. Bilateral posterior vitreous detachment after electroconvulsive therapy. Gen Hosp Psychiatry 2009;31(4):385–7.

88. Grover S, Hazari N, Kate N. Combined use of clozapine and ECT: a review. Acta Neuropsychiatr 2015;27(3):131–42.

89. Munk-Olsen T, Laursen TM, Videbech P, et al. All–cause mortality among recipients of electroconvulsive therapy. Br J Psychiatry 2007;190(5):435–9.
90. Philibert RA, Richards L, Lynch CF, et al. Effect of ECT on mortality and clinical outcome in geriatric unipolar depression. J Clin Psychiatry 1995;56(9):390–4.
91. Wagner KJ, Möllenberg O, Rentrop M, et al. Guide to anaesthetic selection for electroconvulsive therapy. CNS Drugs 2005;19(9):745–58.

Index

Note: Page numbers of article titles are in **boldface** type.

Psychiatr Clin N Am 39 (2016) 531–540
http://dx.doi.org/10.1016/S0193-953X(16)30035-1
0193-953X/16/$ – see front matter

psych.theclinics.com

Moving?

Make sure your subscription moves with you!

To notify us of your new address, find your **Clinics Account Number** (located on your mailing label above your name), and contact customer service at:

Email: journalscustomerservice-usa@elsevier.com

800-654-2452 (subscribers in the U.S. & Canada)
314-447-8871 (subscribers outside of the U.S. & Canada)

Fax number: 314-447-8029

Elsevier Health Sciences Division
Subscription Customer Service
3251 Riverport Lane
Maryland Heights, MO 63043

*To ensure uninterrupted delivery of your subscription, please notify us at least 4 weeks in advance of move.

Printed and bound by CPI Group (UK) Ltd, Croydon, CR0 4YY
08/05/2025
01864686-0006